Who Cares?
The Great British Health Debate

Oliver Morgan

RADCLIFFE MEDICAL PRESS

Radcliffe Medical Press Ltd
18 Marcham Road, Abingdon, Oxon OX14 1AA, UK

British Library Cataloguing in Publication Data

A catalogue record for this book is available from the British Library.

ISBN 1 85775 243 0

Library of Congress Cataloging-in-Publication Data is available.

Typeset by Acorn Bookwork, Salisbury, Wiltshire.
Printed and bound by Biddles Ltd, Guildford and King's Lynn

Contents

Preface

As a nation there are few institutions we care more about than our health service. We are born into it, it is there throughout our lives and we die in its care. It is a peculiarly British creation, created by our own breed of socialists to make sure no one who could not afford health care went without. Unlike other systems around the world, it is still funded mostly by tax and still derives its justification from providing care free at the point of use, according to need. British people still believe the NHS is a defining pillar of their civility.

However, as the service passes through its fiftieth birthday, there is a growing fear that the foundations on which it was established are crumbling. Can a nation which only elects governments that pledge to cut taxes expect to have a fully funded national health service free to everyone who needs it? Or would it be better to abandon what many argue is already the pretence of universalism for a more clear cut system which clearly defines a limit as to what the state will provide? In short, has Britain changed so much in the 50 years since the creation of the NHS that it no longer recognizes the values that underpinned its creation? Until now there have been no radical solutions to these growing problems. Indeed, the attempts to reform the NHS have at worse threatened it and at best, as in the latest series of attempts, prolonged an inevitable national agony.

Meanwhile, the public debate is constrained by the idealism and affection we still hold for the NHS. Arguments focus on short-term issues – closure of hospitals, cuts in local services, tragic though these may be to people involved. Against this background, risk-averse politicians shy away from taking decisive steps to save the system. This book looks behind the headlines and explains in a simple, straightforward way what has happened to our NHS and what future waits in store. It is intended to be read by anyone who reads a newspaper of whatever shape or size.

There are several things however it does not set out to do. It does not tackle detailed medical or technical questions and does not, unfortunately, deal with the problems of mental illness and care in the community. It focuses on the relationship between the primary and hospital sectors of the NHS, the private sector, the managers and politicians that run them and the public that use them. I hope that, despite any omissions, it provides a readable and stimulating account for health professionals and laymen alike.

Oliver Morgan
January 1998

Acknowledgements

I would like to thank the many people who generously gave up their valuable time while I was researching and writing this book. I cannot mention all of them by name because there are too many, and many also spoke to me on an unattributable basis.

I should like to thank David Sinclair, my editor at the *Financial Mail on Sunday*, who commissioned the original series of articles which prompted me to write this book and for his encouragement and advice over the two years it has taken to produce. Roger Hymas and David Bryant of BUPA asked me to write the book and again offered encouragement throughout. In Kate Roxburgh I had an excellent researcher and a combative and testing sparring partner to whom I am grateful for telling me what I was trying to say.

Roderick Nye, director of the Social Market Foundation and Perri 6, research director of Demos, have both provided extremely valuable insights into different aspects of the making of health policy, as have a number of policy makers and advisors. I am grateful to Greg Clark and Tony Hockley for their frequently sought advice.

I owe particular thanks to Frank Honigsbaum of Birmingham University and Kingsley Manning of Newchurch both of whom generously gave up a lot of time to read a very long first draft and offered detailed and incisive comments. The King's Fund's Peter Griffiths and Sir Duncan Nichol also met me on several occasions for interviews and advice.

Gillian Nineham at Radcliffe Medical Press acted as a sure handed, ruthless but always constructive editor and Jamie Etherington was helpful throughout the later stages.

Any errors of fact or of judgement remain my own.

Finally, I would like to thank my wife, Charlotte, for putting up with me while she gave birth to two children.

For Charlotte and Benedict

1 Big sister is watching you: the future of the National Health Service

Imagine you have a new-born daughter. In 2048, the year the National Health Service is 100, she will be 50. But what kind of a service will it be, if it is there at all? That may not be a question you feel you can easily answer – any more than you can predict whether your child will be a sculptress, nurse, prime minister or Olympic 100 metre hurdler. What kind of service would you like it to be? What will children born this year inherit?

In half a century's time the capabilities of medicine will be awesome. Doctors will have at their disposal technologies that now seem pure science fiction. If your daughter needed a major operation, the options would be myriad. What is more, it could be she who would choose what to have done to her, where and when it would be done and by whom, all in the full knowledge of how much it would cost and how it would be paid for.

The British health care system could be a smooth, seamless range of services, with diagnosis and monitoring, emergency care and major surgery, community services and public health all linked into a computerized system. It could be different from the compartmentalized medical profession of today, where the consultant's hospital is his castle and the family doctor may work from a poky lock-up surgery or run-down community health centre. The caring profession could be a far more unified organization, with teams of doctors and nurses working together in big hospitals, community medicentres and your home. They could be plugged into an international information system in which their availability and areas of interest would be accessible to and summonable by all at the touch of a button.

Say your daughter needed a hip replacement in 2048. Today doctors see replacing hips as a routine operation. For patients, however, it is often anything but. Last autumn, to have had a hip operation carried out on the NHS you would have had to have waited between 14 weeks (if you live in Bridgend) and 5.5 years (in Cambridgeshire) to have the operation.[a] You will wait for an initial outpatient appointment for six weeks or more, and then you will wait for months until a slot becomes available for the actual operation. You will have little say over who does the surgery, where it is done, or at what time of day. When you reach the hospital, geared up and mentally prepared for the pain of being cut open and stitched up again, you could find you are sent home because operating theatre space is needed to deal with an emergency. Back you go into the queue, to another month or more of pain and anxiety. If you want to jump the queue you either have to pay out some £3500, or be one of the six million people in Britain who have private health insurance. Then, although it could be the very same doctor who sees you at the outpatient appointment and carries out the replacement, it is a matter of weeks from beginning to end.

But for the majority of people who do not have this option – your daughter, for instance – the future may be brighter. Your daughter will be in a much better position to decide the nature of her treatment herself. She will enter a system where consultation, diagnosis, treatment and aftercare are systematically and efficiently monitored by computer. She will e-mail her NHS local health team – incorporating family medicine specialists, as well as consultants – at the local community health centre. She will book an appointment. A reply will be waiting in her own e-mail box when she returns from her job at the end of the day, suggesting a number of dates, and requesting a brief summary of her symptoms and her thoughts on diagnosis – if she is able to provide them.

Your daughter uses her home computer to help understand what has happened to her. She leads a busy life and rarely sees the doctor. However, she has mentioned an ache in her thigh to him before. The ache has grown worse and worse, and now presents itself as a wrenching pain when she climbs the stairs, and keeps her awake at nights if she has done a lot of walking during the day. She suspects it might be arthritis, but is not sure. She enters the Internet.

She downloads her medical records from the health smart card, which she carries in her wallet, on to her computer. She then moves into the healthweb and a number of options appear – grouped into two categories – arthritic and muscular problems. She is then able to refer to a database of medical literature to investigate further, moving between summaries of academic work prepared by the Patients Association, and more detailed accounts of conditions and possible treatments, from injections to cure muscle pain to hip replacement for severe arthritis. She does not come to any conclusion but types what she feels each day, and what she has learned from the material she has read into a pre-prepared diagnostic

---

[a] National waiting list helpline

questionnaire – could it be muscle pain, or is it arthritis? She sends the questionnaire, along with her chosen appointment date, back to the health centre.

On the day of her appointment she talks to her general health adviser (GHA) – as the family doctor is by then known, explaining her symptoms in detail, informing him of what she has read on the healthweb. The GHA has already checked her medical records on his password-protected database, and recognizes the growing leg pains as a problem dating back three years. He believes the symptoms point to arthritis. He does two things. First he requests an appointment with a specialist. He asks your daughter which specialist she would like to use. There is a list of ortho-paedic surgeons around Britain specializing in exactly the symptoms shown by your daughter. They are classified according to where they work, years' experience, ability and availability. The ability score shows how many specific operations are carried out and how many of those have complications.

Along with the GHA your daughter clicks on the screen to get behind the statistics, discovering the seriousness and difficulty of the operations that each surgeon carried out, and the diagnostic characteristics of the group of patients. She decides on her specialist – choosing the best surgeon who is available for her condition at the time she wants. She chooses one who lives 400 miles away in Scotland. The GHA then dispatches the request through the computer, using the same integrated system that your daughter used to book her appointment. He takes her through a number of possibilities for treatment to keep the pain at bay. While this is happening the computer at the nearby medicentre is transmitting a request to Scotland for a specialist appointment. At the end of the half-hour consultation your daughter leaves with a guaranteed home appointment with the specialist and a package of pills to relieve her pain.

It is a home appointment with a difference. On the day a nurse from the GHA's practice arrives with a portable scanner. This is linked to her computer. At the appointed time the Scottish specialist comes on-line and uses the scanner to examine the hip joint and surrounding muscles and confirms the diagnosis, simultaneously feeding this into your daughter's medical records. He speaks to your daughter over the telelink. A hip replacement is needed. The appointment is booked: 5 July at 2pm.

At exactly 2pm on 5 July the operation starts. It is undertaken in a 10-bedded medical centre a mile from your daughter's home by a high-tech. robot.

Anaesthetic and monitoring are carried out by the nurse and a highly trained team of technicians, with a televised link to a specialist in a major hospital 50 miles away should advice be required. If there are complications – a blood clot, for example – the nurses will be well trained to meet them and will be advised over the link. The operation will take a fraction of the time it would take today and be carried out with a steadier hand and with greater accuracy than is possible at present. If you could watch it happening you would be astonished.

Your daughter is first anaesthetized by the nurse. She is then taken to the operating theatre, where the operating table is crowned by a series of metal arms, each fitted with the precise surgical tools needed for the operation. This robot makes an incision in her hip using a scalpel. Her thigh is held in place by one arm, while another removes the head of the femur – the hip bone – which is diseased with arthritis. The robot then has to fit the artificial hip, known as the prosthetic, in its place. First the robot grinds out a hole in the bone into which it can fit the prosthetic. An arm with a milling tool moves in to create the space, operating within an accuracy of half a millimetre. When this has been done the robot fits the hip replacement, sliding the spike-shaped tongue of the artificial joint into the top of the femur by exerting strong pressure in a series of minute bursts without having to knock it into place with a hammer. The risk of a fracture is lessened. Once the shining metal ball joint is in place the robot manipulates it back into the socket, and begins the process of stitching back tissue and skin.[1]

It would seem to you at the bedside that the operation was being done without human involvement at all, save the team of nurses fitting and removing implements from the robots arms, cleaning and sterilizing equipment as it was used, and monitoring progress, ready to intervene in the event of a problem.

By 2048 this may well be possible. But it may not necessarily be acceptable – a human at the other end of the line may be demanded, thus the surgeon in Scotland. Every move the robot makes is monitored by the surgeon. The technology used to link him to events in the operating theatre dwarfs the capabilities of the robot. The surgeon is linked via satellite in real time to three-dimensional images of your daughter. The robot is also linked to a computer and, like the doctor, can see inside her leg to the bone by computer imaging. A sensor on the tools allows the surgeon to monitor progress. On his three-dimensional display he will see exact video images of the leg and thigh bone, but these will be combined with the computer images to 'see through' tissue to the bone.

Every second the surgeon is precisely aware of where the robot implements are in relation to your daughter's body – to arteries, veins and ligaments – so it does not stray and cause bleeding. As he moves his head, and as she moves throughout the operation, the system adjusts. The robot uses information from the computer imager to grind out the bone and carry out the operation, while another computer checks that the robot is making the right movements. At all times, the surgeon is aware of what is happening.

Your daughter is allowed to go home within a couple of hours of the operation. If she feels more comfortable, or if there are problems that need close observation, she can stay overnight in the patient hotel facilities next to the medicentre. Either way, she will need a great deal of care to manage the pain of the operation, ensure that any complications are dealt with and that she is not left feeling isolated. Home will be a rather different place from the home of today. The computer system she and the doctors used as the fulcrum of the diagnostic and medical process now becomes a telecare manager. The home is converted temporarily into a hospital. It is linked to the medicentre, where the nurses are able to keep track of your daughter's recovery and progress on-line. To begin with a great deal of care will be needed and the 24-hour team of nurses visits the home regularly to help, for example, with meals, washing and managing pain.[2]

As the wound heals and your daughter regains mobility, the computer takes over. The telecare system linked to a number of video points and sensors in your daughter's home allows the nursing team to monitor her movement around the home – when she last visited the toilet, when she last took her medication, when she last used the kitchen – and they are instantly contactable. It also allows your daughter to monitor her recovery – to understand how her wound is healing, to check heart rate and blood flow. In case of emergency a team of paramedics is on five minute standby from a moving mobile centre, with fast access up the ladder of care centres – the GHA's health centre, the medicentre, and in case of life-threatening complications, to the highly specialized super hospital some 50 miles away, linked into the on-line system and staffed with a 24-hour accident and emergency unit.

As your daughter heals and begins to walk normally once more, the centre of care moves again – back to the GHA's medicentre, where she attends group physiotherapy sessions and is helped to rejoin the normal pace of life.

She will even know the exact cost of her operation because the amount will be on her next pay slip. The figure will be marked down next to the amount of income tax paid into the NHS. It will not be added as a payment to her tax bill; it will be there to show how much has been spent against how much has been paid in for 2048. Two other figures relating to the NHS will also be printed there – the total amount paid into the NHS through income tax since the Government agreed to dedicate a proportion of tax to the NHS in 2010, and the total amount she has cost the service since then. She will be able to see at a glance what the NHS has done for her.

The mechanisms for payment will also be easy to follow. Your daughter's GHA will have been involved in drawing up detailed plans for the needs of his patients in conjunction with the local health partnership commissioning group – the health authority of twenty-first century Britain.

The number of people requiring hip replacements will have been estimated along with the hundreds of other requirements and treatments making up the health services needed in the area. Age patterns, historic need, technological development all channelled through sophisticated computer models will have allowed the GHA, along with the authority, to come up with a clear idea of what will be needed on both an annual and longer term basis, and a budget will have been paid out to the health authority, part of which will have put it into an isolated GHA fund. All of this information will be available on computer in a simple format so that your daughter will be able to fit what she has used into the general pattern. She will also be able to see how the authority's money is spent year by year.

So, if your daughter did need a hip replacement in 2048, this could well be the kind of system you would like to see in place. This all supposes, of course, that she lives alone. With a husband, children, or even you to look after her, her convalescence will be a less isolating experience. But the telecare system will still be there.

A National Health Service, however, amounts to more than 'elective' surgery for long-term conditions such as arthritis. You will want to know that there will be top quality emergency facilities available within the shortest possible time if your daughter has an accident. Despite the time factor, the system could be computerized and managed to be as flexible as the non-emergency care services she would need for her hip replacement.

The number and size of medical establishments in 2048 could be very different from today. There would be a diverse range of local centres starting with the home, with its computerized telecare and telemedicine linkups, allowing the NHS to go to your daughter rather than vice versa. Next up would be the GHA's health centre, where uncomplicated procedures – plastic surgery, excision of lumps – is carried out, where physiotherapy, osteopathy, chiropractice, homeopathy and other services are based, where outpatient clinics are held by specialist doctors, and where there is day-to-day contact between patients and the NHS. Then there would be a smaller number of medicentres like the one in which your daughter had her operation – perhaps one per every 50 000 people. At the top of the pyramid there would be a smaller number of highly specialized hospitals where complex treatments are carried out and where accident and emergency services are based.[3]

The crucial question is: 'if your daughter had an accident, could you rely on this system?' The super hospital with its emergency department backed up by specialists such as neurosurgeons, cardiologists, and trauma orthopaedic consultants may be a lot further away than the district general hospital is from you at present. The GHA and medicentre services may be better for some needs, and may – even by 2048 – be able to deal with some serious accidents quickly. They will, however, need quick access to specialist emergency care quickly in the event of unpredictable complications and they will not be able to deal with major accidents. Major trauma centres will be needed.[4]

From the moment accidents happen the clock starts ticking. There is a belief in a 'golden hour' when the chances of survival from a serious injury are highest, so time is critical. The ambulance that is by your daughter's side within five minutes is a different vehicle from the one with which we are familiar. It will be a mobile emergency unit, complete with electrocardiogram, scanning equipment and a full range of emergency treatments. It will have three specialist level paramedics on board who are able quickly to assess her condition, staunch bleeding, check internal organs and brain activity and give immediate emergency care. The ambulance is also linked into the healthweb.

Accident and emergency consultants are available to advise the team as they race to the hospital. As the paramedics work, a third member of the team assesses availability of beds in various facilities at varying distances. If major treatment is needed the driver will go to the trauma centre, some 50 miles away. If less complex treatment is needed the driver will go to a medicentre closer by. He also relays regular updates on your daughter's condition to the centre to allow its staff to access her medical records and prepare treatment for when she arrives. Despite the fastest and most sure-footed response by paramedics, your daughter may still not survive. However, the existence of rapid-response units is essential for a service that reassures the public that everything will be done to keep them alive – and to maintain faith in the health care system. It is the least you can expect for your children.

Here and now

This brave new world of health care is not all fantasy. In fact, in the Autumn of 1997 the Government promised something similar within ten years. The technology to create such an integrated 'space age' system is here or hereabouts. Medical research, for example, is being put on-line – available to patients now. The implications in 50 years' time are enormous

– patients could challenge diagnosis and treatment. Hopefully this would only occur in extreme cases – the growing knowledge of the patient could be used to more productive effect to forge a new relationship with doctors.

Monitoring and administering care in the home is coming about too. 'Hospital at Home' (HAH) schemes are up and running around the country – the most well known is in Peterborough where a nurse bank is used to provide 24-hour cover and to keep people out of their local hospitals by allowing them to stay in their own homes. It is used mostly to care for elderly patients with cancer or suffering from stroke, but the principle is being broadened. Hospital at Home schemes cover both long-term care for elderly people in their homes and acute care for people who have come out of hospital and are expected to recover soon afterwards. Work by telecommunications companies into telecare systems is increasing the opportunities for bringing increasingly sophisticated monitoring by nurses and patients in the home closer, as well as linking hospitals around the country to allow services like ultrasound scanning to be shared by hospitals hundreds of miles apart.[5]

Scientists are on the threshold of creating the technology to carry out robotic operations, spearheaded by the need for high tech. systems for military use. Trials on a system that could perform exactly such an operation have been carried out in Sacramento, California, by IBM. In fact, in the case of hip replacements, the technology is already so advanced as to make the orthopaedic surgeon redundant in less than 50 years' time.[1]

Surgery itself is already becoming less violent. Endoscopes allow doctors to send surgical tools voyaging into the body through small holes in the skin instead of making large incisions, manipulating them via optic fibres while viewing a video monitor. Lithotripters use shock waves to pulverise gall and kidney stones, lasers can be used for cancers and treatment of coronary heart disease, and new drugs attack new conditions and can be taken for pregnancy termination where formerly surgical procedures were required. The ideal of 'trackless surgery' – where surgeons can attack malignant cells in the body without wounding the patient in the process – is coming closer. Hand-held, pencil-shaped lamps, costing £10 000 to £15 000 can, for example, be used to kill off malignant cancer cells by activating a light sensitive drug soaked into the skin, while the patient sits comfortably in the doctor's surgery.[1,6]

Diagnosis using scanning equipment is already advanced. With computerized tomography and magnetic resonance imaging, a three-dimensional picture of the body can be built up using a series of minute cross sections to create three-dimensional, see-through pictures of organs, bones, blood vessels and tissues. These technologies are the basis for harnessing imaging equipment to allow robotic surgery.

Transplant technology is driving forward, and anti-rejection drugs are widening the horizons and the now-familiar repertoire of possibilities. Artificial components are becoming more sophisticated and widespread. The pacemaker has been superseded by the electronic heart, wired into the body to help the real heart regenerate itself. The aim is eventually to remove the device after the real organ has regrown.[7]

Nor is research limited to the high tech. New applications for old technology are constantly being found. The perennial favourite is aspirin, invented as a painkiller, but now recognized as a preventative for heart disease and, most recently, a treatment to stop miscarriage. Doctors at Guy's and St Thomas's hospitals in London last year found the birth rate in women with Hughes Syndrome – which causes blood clots leading to miscarriage – was increased from 19% to 70%, and believe other women who have difficulties giving birth could benefit from the treatment as well.[8] Research extends even further back – to a renewed interest in pre-industrial purges like leaches and maggots.

Just as new uses for the age-old aspirin are constantly being found, so medical science is discovering new ways of tackling formerly untreatable problems. Understanding the human genome – the structure made up of the millions of individual genes which form the blueprint of who we are – and of deoxyribonucleic acid (DNA), which forms the building blocks of life is creating a new biotechnology industry. Your daughter could well be dependent on it for a range of treatments in the next millennium. It can help in diagnosing conditions by cloning antibodies – the body's self-protection system – which can detect the existence of particular substances accurately. Monoclonal antibodies can detect malignant cancers, hormones and infectious diseases. They can be packaged in formats to make diagnosis easy – increasingly purchased over the counter. Today pregnancy kits are available for testing in the comfort of the home. In 2048 there will be few conditions your daughter will be unable to test for in her home.

Prevention and cure are other areas where biotechnology could revolutionize health care. Genetics has already been used to produce certain substances used within the body, like insulin. The future holds the prospect of loading antibodies with drugs to combat diseases like cancers. The power that such a cure for cancer holds can be shown by the companies that are researching into the treatments. One, Oxford-based British Biotech, reached a share price of £32.65 in 1996 – the highest quote on the stock exchange at the time – and it has not produced a treatment, let alone a profit. When it reported interim findings on research into a cancer drug in 1995 its share price went up five fold. When later reports were pessimistic, the share price plummeted, pulling the industry down too.

Already therapy is producing cures for genetic disorders. The first 'map' of the human genome was produced in France in 1993, and the first steps to actual treatments are being made. A gene that causes cystic fibrosis – a disease that affects salivary, intestinal, pancreatic, lung and gall bladder glands, making them produce a thick mucus – has been discovered, and pioneering treatment has shown some success with sufferers. Doctors have also isolated genes that cause the degenerative Huntingdon's disease – a brain disorder that leads to a loss of nerve cells – and tests are being carried out around the world into cancers. Success so far has been focused on single gene disorders – like cystic fibrosis or Huntingdon's disease. Researchers are confident that by 2048, many diseases your daughter may suffer from could be treated by genetics. From here the possibilities multiply. Your grandchildren could be screened at birth for genetic disorders and either have disease-causing genes removed or be instructed in ways of life that will help them postpone or avoid the onset of conditions to which they are prone. If they are likely to be short, they could be made tall. Brown eyes could be turned blue. A ruddy complexion could be exchanged for a Mediterranean one.

A detailed examination of the state of medical technology and the issues its advances throws up would be a book in themselves, and goes beyond the scope of what can be tackled here. However, some questions are addressed in the pages that follow.

The opportunities for exploiting scientific advance are enormous. But what is the point of all this technology? Is it to pay drug companies millions to search for miracle cures for deadly but rare diseases, to spur geneticists into engineering supermen and women, to give surgeons new toys to play with? Or is it to provide more useful care for patients in the time, place and form of their choosing?

The generation game

With all these options, it may seem as though your child will be spoilt for choice. Certainly, that is how those who were 50 when the NHS was created would phrase it. At that time, anything provided by the State to its people, exhausted after six years of war, was a sign of benevolence and the triumph of humanity over want. In the post-war years to question what was provided by the service was like Oliver Twist asking for more.

But we no longer see ourselves as passive patients being operated on, we want the same service from the NHS as we get in Sainsbury's. That the hospital is part of a health market is now a reality, if an imperfect and crude one. The motors of markets are choice and competition. The war-shattered nation that witnessed the creation of the Welfare State would not recognize it now, and might well wonder at what has happened to the values of civility and serenity its creator, Aneurin Bevan, used to describe as the spirit behind the NHS. Bevan, however, was a man of his time. Our children are likely to be more demanding consumers of everything from toothpaste to hip replacements and electronic hearts than we are.[1,9]

Your future

It is time to ask yourself where you will be in 2048. You may well be alive, in your eighties. Whether you will be alive and well has a lot to do with how you decide to live. The high technology NHS will help you if you need urgent treatment, but finding fulfilment into the later years of life will rely more on how you live your life to keep you free from the need for care. The importance of the prevention of illness over cure has been recognized in the Health of the Nation strategy, which aimed to 'add years to life and add life to years' by targeting key areas of ill health – to begin with heart disease and stroke, cancer, mental illness, HIV and AIDS and accidents.[10] The strategy aims – but does not always succeed – to increase public awareness of issues causing these diseases and to keep people from needing treatment to cure them. The new Government has set new lower, wider targets, aiming to reinvigorate what was seen as an ineffective campaign.

Ever more information will be available to you over the computerized channels and through the media on what to eat, when to exercise, and public policies will be tied ever more to promoting health. The newly created Minister for Public Health should become the axis around which government departments are forced into thinking about the health aspects of their policies, and this could feed into more localized action. The idea of healthy cities, first promoted by the World Health Organization in 1986 could catch on around Britain, allowing the goals of cleanliness, community action and involvement, an abundance of healthy activities, high employment levels and institutions to promote health and healthy living to be reached. Local environmental, educational, trade, industrial, transport and health bodies could be linked in with the NHS to allow GHAs to work alongside them in providing advice and support on how to live healthily and on how to keep yourself the right side of targets like those set out in 'Health of the Nation'.

Public health in the brave new world into which you and your children are heading is as important as the other highly technical treatment side. Should you fall ill with the chronic heart and vascular diseases like stroke that continue to dominate the horizons of the NHS in the future, you will be able to plug into the Hospital at Home schemes described above, or fall into the long-term nursing care safety net that will be available for you in 2048. This should happen only after the health system has done its best to keep you well. Both prevention and cure should come together to form a whole service capable of keeping people healthier and treating them quickly and effectively if they fall ill. Efficient and precise management between the various agencies that provide care is as important in achieving this scenario as the astonishing advances in medical technology being made around the world.

But this vision of a healthy new world we have outlined poses a great challenge to today's health system for it encapsulates the three classic demand pressures building up to crack the ability of Britain's NHS to survive its second 50 years: the ageing of the population, the costs of technology and the rise in consumer expectations. The health service claims it needs 3% growth in its annual budget to survive today's demand pressures. The future could be bleaker. This doomsday scenario has led a number of studies into the future of the NHS to conclude that private medical insurance is the only way in which an increasing funding gap will be met. Chief among these was a report by *Healthcare 2000* in Autumn 1995, which sketched a future in which the demand on health care increased while the resources to pay for it diminished as tax cutting became a political way of life. That report pointed to the need to increase private sector provision to fill the gap. Indeed, the radical health service reforms, planned by the Thatcher government in the 1980s were prompted by similar readings of the future.[11]

First, the very fact that you are more likely than your parents to reach your eighties will place a greater burden on health services. The causes of death have changed dramatically this century. Death from infectious disease has fallen steeply, matched by an equally sharp rise in long-term illness like heart disease, stroke and cancer. The population is ageing. There are currently 9 million people aged over 65. By 2036 the number is projected to be 15 million. But it is today's 30 years olds – the parents of tomorrow's children – for whom the most dramatic change is expected. According to policy analysts Laing & Buisson in 1994 there were 1.009 million people aged over 85 in Britain, 1.7% of the population. The number in 2050 is calculated to be 2.7 million, 4.8% of the population.[12] The proportion of old people to young will grow. The changing nature of society, with women going out to work instead of fulfilling the 'traditional' caring role is also portrayed as driving up costs because what was once provided as a free service by the family – will be provided by paid carers and financed by the taxpayer. Coupled with the upwards trend in chronic disease, the resource implications for the health service pose serious questions.

The cost of technology is another problem. The robosurgery, computer link-ups, paramedic teams and scanning services that characterized the system outlined at the beginning of this chapter are often portrayed as driving costs up, and indeed such technologies are not cheap. There are an increasing number of drugs to treat hitherto untreatable conditions and they are also expensive. The Beta interferon group of drugs to treat multiple sclerosis is the most well-known and controversial. It is difficult to come up with an exact figure on the increase in spending caused by technology but a Department of Health estimate built into Government spending calculations puts it at a 0.5% increase in total expenditure each year.[10]

On top of these assumptions comes the Sainsbury's factor. Instead of a cowed silence in the family doctor's surgery, you will boldly surf the Internet to arrive at your own conclusions and demand treatment. This will cost money. Demands for better services create pressures because money is needed to meet them. Intolerance with waiting lists caused the former Health Secretary, Virginia Bottomley, to launch a national waiting-list initiative, aimed at cutting waiting-list times. This was at a time when the annual increases in the Health Service budget were in line with the 3% needed to stop the system grinding to a halt. But, as we shall see in later chapters, focusing on waiting lists, viewed by politicians as a soft option for budgetary cuts, took attention away from other areas of the system, which found resources stretched. Expectations of a better, more consumer-friendly service took their toll.

However, the case that the system will collapse under the burden of spiralling demand is not conclusive. The frequently used phrase 'infinite demand' is controversial – many argue no one needs all the services provided by the NHS throughout their life. Matching it with supply is harder. Commentators have argued that people may live longer but that they may also remain healthier for longer. They may not use the resources of the Health Service until the final period of their lives, which may be no more prolonged than it is today. In addition the kind of care needed by those people who are ill is generally low tech. and therefore less expensive. Studies of countries with different population profiles have also concluded that ageing populations do not necessarily cause higher costs.

Stephen Dorrell's White Paper of November 1996 stated:

the rate of increase in the numbers of very elderly people is now slowing down. Between 1986 and 1996 there were 302 000 additional people aged 85 and above. Between 2006–2016 that falls to 100000, although it rises again to 153000 from 2016 to 2026 ... It would be wrong to assume unmanageable pressures.[13]

Costs imposed by ageing people are not necessarily borne by the NHS. The costs of long-term care are now borne by the social services departments of local authorities. These are means tested, with payment expected from those with assets over £16000. The notion of a free service for all is therefore part of history for those in need of long-term care but individuals are meeting the costs. Who knows which way local administration of health services will go in 50 years time?

These factors have led a recent study to conclude:

Undoubtedly additional resources will be required in certain areas of care for the elderly. However, this does not mean that demographic change will lead to insurmountable problems for the NHS or exacerbate the priority setting process. After all if the NHS was able to survive a previous major demographic change (the baby boom) there is every reason to believe it can do so again.[14]

Even if high-tech. care proliferates there are those who argue that it will not necessarily drive up costs. Some technologies produce results that cost more – keeping people alive longer, but not making them independent of the need for care. Treatments for cancer clearly illustrate this. Others produce results that reduce the burden on other parts of health care resources. Zantac is an example. The idea of a 0.5% annual increase in costs is consistently challenged by those who point to other industries, for example computing, where technology has enhanced quality and driven costs down over time. More research is needed into the effects of technology before bold assertions that it will drive the NHS beyond our grasp can be accepted. In addition, Government control over health spending and consumer responsibility are cited as forces for cost-containment.[14]

Studies show that while heart bypass surgery may greatly increase the demand for medical services, many drug treatments can reduce them. For example the number of 'finished consultant episodes' – the measure of activity by doctors in the NHS – involving heart bypasses went up from 9655 in 1988/89 to 16047 in 1993/94. The increased workload should mean the cost of each operation could come down, but the total cost will be higher. Technology can also create innovation in the location of care. Treatment can be shifted out of expensive hospitals into communities, into the home.

As for public expectation, the key is information, and high-quality information. With details of treatments should come details of their costs. If information on what medicine can do is made widely available, it must be accompanied by what medicine costs. Patients are currently largely ignorant about costs in the NHS, so it is unclear what effect the knowledge of cost would have on them if they had choices of treatment presented to them. Breaking the notion that health is a 'free good' – which it is not, because it is only available free at the point of demand – may have important consequences on the way we use services.

These arguments were also favoured by the Conservative government, which in Autumn 1996 dismissed demographic, technological and expectation-led demands in its White Paper, which included a foreword by the former Prime Minister in which he argued that the NHS was 'part of Britain ... it must continue to be there when we need it.' Even Sir Duncan Nichol, former Chief Executive of the NHS Executive and one of the authors of the controversial *Healthcare 2000* report admits: 'I am changing my mind.'[15]

It is clear, then, that there is controversy over visions of the future. Indeed, the *Healthcare 2000* report was dismissed when it came out in September 1995 as being funded by drug companies, taking the view only of the private sector in suggesting that the NHS is not up to the job. Deciding on where the truth lies between the two extremes is difficult. What is more than likely, however, is that the system will face greater pressure in future. Demand is likely to outstrip whatever increases in spending the health system attracts and whatever efficiencies it manages to make to allow that money to go further. Those who argue against the *Healthcare 2000* prognosis admit this much, claiming that the system has dealt with similar swells of demand in the past, and will continue to be able to do so in future. The question is how. The doomsday theorists can find support for their view in what has happened to long-term care for the elderly – the NHS has scaled down its involvement in the system over many years, the private sector has stepped in to fill the gap, and 'partnership' proposals, which amount to a subsidy to private sector insurers, are being considered. But other interpretations would point out that partnership schemes are pragmatic ways of solving the NHS dilemma – asking those who can afford it to contribute without paying at the point of use, while keeping a national system for those who cannot.

In the view of many health professionals and some academics the answer to these problems is simple: we should spend more on the NHS. The British Medical Association (BMA) – the trade body representing doctors – in 1996 said the NHS would hit a serious funding crisis unless an extra £6 billion was pumped into the service. Doctors were deserting the NHS because of the long hours they were working and Dr Sandy Macara, the chairman of the BMA said: 'We cannot go on doing more and more work for more and more patients with less and less resources.'

He added: 'Individuals, like structures such as the NHS, can sustain only so much stress before they collapse from exhaustion.'[16] In the summer of 1997, the BMA claimed the system needed an extra £1 billion a year over the next five years to avert crisis, and said it is reserving judgement on the new Government.

In fact, the proportion of gross domestic product (GDP) spent on health in Britain has risen in recent years, due, to some degree, to the huge costs imposed on the NHS by the latest round of reforms in the system. Spending on the NHS for 1996/97 was £42.3 billion, some 6.5% of GDP. This figure compares with cash sums of £16.3 billion in 1984, £27.9 billion in 1990, and £39.8 million in 1994. To these figures need to be added the cost of other elements in the health system, including private health care, which brings the total up to some 7.1% of GDP. This is up from 6.9% between 1993 and 1995 and 5.8% in 1988. In cash terms, spending on the entire health system has risen from £27.3 billion in 1988 to more than £50 billion today – which includes spending on private treatment. The cash figures do not, however, take into account inflation: either the general measure of the retail price index, or medical inflation, which is higher because the goods and services the health system buys – largely composed of wages, which rise faster than prices, and high-cost technology – rise more quickly in price than other goods and services. In total spending on the health system – not just the NHS – spending in 1990 was £32.998 million. In constant prices taking inflation into account, the level rose to £36.07 million in 1994.[17]

Nevertheless, by whatever measure, other countries do spend more on health care. The US, for example, spent 11.5% of GDP on health in 1988, rising to 14.5% last year, France 8.6% and 9.9%, Germany 8.8% and 9.6%, The Netherlands 8.1% and 8.8%, Japan 6.8% and 7.2%. We British do not spend as much on health as the rest of the world.[18] The problem for the UK, wedded to universal state care, is that the deficit in Europe and America is made up with private medicine.

But demand for health care is, if not infinite, so large that any increase in funding will simply uncover more unmet demand. We could spend double or more of our national income on health and still not meet all the need.

Today's dilemmas

The challenges of the future confront a system that is trapped in the past. It is 50 years since Aneurin Bevan oversaw the foundation of the NHS and set in train the relationships within the service and between it and the private sector. But the paradox of the NHS is that although it was planned and sold in the spirit of technological advance and progressive rational planning its main characteristics have remained preserved in aspic. There has been much noisy reform, but little progress on the fundamental issues.

The noise of reform is a symptom of this lack of change. Each development to the system has been controversial as the ultra-conservative interest groups within that system campaign to block change. Perhaps conservatism is a function of health because people fear change to a system that is there to protect them from fear itself.

Indeed Bevan's famous statement that the NHS was there not just to provide medical help but spiritual comfort can also be seen as a retrenchment clause. He said: 'society becomes more wholesome, more serene, and spiritually healthier, if it knows that its citizens have at the back of their consciousness the knowledge that not only themselves, but all their fellows have access, when ill, to the best that medical skill can provide'.[19]

There is a neat symmetry in the timing of the system's 50th anniversary. It was created in the wake of a Labour landslide in 1945, alongside the other great columns of the Welfare State: social security, and the education service. Fifty years on, Labour has the second of its great twentieth-century landslides. It is planning a radical overhaul both of the education and social security systems, but it is not doing so for health, which is arguably in as difficult a position as social security, and perhaps worse off than education. However, the funding pressures that face the British health system over the next 50 years will need radical thought if it is to remain effective and be perceived as such.

The fundamental problems with health have been clear since before the foundation of the NHS and, as I shall argue in Chapter 2, they were in fact institutionalized in its foundation: the dominance of the medical model of health, the dominance of the medical profession, the subordination of managers, the deafness of the system to its users, the lack of information and clarity, the requirement to ration and to hide rationing, the inflexibility of provision of health care through the hospital and the acceptance and maintenance of traditional medical training and professional practices.

The interest groups within the system: doctors, politicians, users, managers, all have separate interests and have a desire to see these arrangements maintained. Although there are clear and pressing economic, financial and managerial problems the political economy of the system limits the capacity for reform to make it function better.

It is here that a central theme of the book emerges. The service was founded, in Rudolf Klein's words, in a spirit of scientific rationalism. But we do not have what the great epidemiologist Archie Cochrane called a rational national health service because of the interest groups it contains. This book takes a thematic look at the problems facing the Government.

In the next chapter I shall outline the development of medicine, the medical profession, the hospital system and the foundation of the NHS, arguing that the pressures built into the system in 1948 were the result of centuries-old attitudes and customs. The remaining chapters will attempt to anatomize these forces and analyse them.

The spirit of rationalism underpinned the internal market reforms introduced from 1990. Fundamentally these were a supply-side answer to a demand-side problem. Although they attempted to control demand by altering peoples' behaviour and the way they used the service, they left unanswered the key question – do we spend enough on health? The market itself fails on a number of levels. First it was the wrong metaphor to choose for what needed to be done, and what in effect was achieved. Economic theory tells us that free markets in health care fail because individuals mostly have too little information and are faced with catastrophe which undermine their informed choice-making power, and because insurance organizations tend to insure only young healthy people, while the elderly are left vulnerable. This, as we shall see, places great tension on the relationship between doctors and patients. Mounting a fundamental reform on a word with these associations, albeit qualified with the addition of 'internal'.

But the failure of reform was practical as well as theoretical. The system clarified a number of key problems that needed – and still need – solving. It was able to do this by creating an analytical framework with which to view the system – the purchaser/provider split. With purchasers analysing and demanding greater efficiencies from providers who were bound to hit targets, systemic obstructions became evident. Doctors were unaccountable. There was no clear link between what was spent and what was delivered by the system. The hospital network was inefficient. The need to ration care implicitly was stifling discussion about how funds should be spent.

So the real failure of market reform is paradoxical. By creating the purchaser/provider split it has rationally identified what needs solving. However, the association with markets suggested that the end results would be a lot more radical than they needed – and turned out – to be. On top of this was a series of structural weaknesses in the internal market which distorted the system.

In addition to this was a political failure. Past governments have been unable to sell the changes to the public, and unwilling to try, instead concentrating on constantly legitimizing the creation of the internal market itself in the teeth of opposition assault on the inappropriateness of market 'ideology' or 'dogma' in health.

The result has been political defensiveness and sterile policy. Labour in opposition played an equally important part, and this points to a further paradox. On the face of it, Labour has attacked the internal market, pointing to consequences it claimed the market would create – the destruction of the NHS through fragmentation, inequity, cost and privatization. But, because of political intervention, it did not create them.

For the new Government to meet the challenges presented by health policy it needs both new courage and new vision. Until recently it has been ideologically opposed to markets in all areas of economic life, arguing that they cost jobs and concentrate wealth in the hands of rich capitalists. The new administration has, however, accepted the value of markets in business life. It has not allowed itself to do so yet in social policy – at least in public.

Instead the internal market has been used as a stick to beat the Conservatives in public. But the political noise from Labour may hide a nasty truth – it has no better ideas of its own.

If Labour continues its attack on the internal market because of its ideological opposition by sweeping it away, it could also undo many positive developments of the last ten years. Instead, it is vital that there is a positive evaluation of why the internal market failed and a search for ways of making acceptable the necessary changes it pointed towards – increased accountability, a rational hospital network and so on – by creating an acceptable, alternative mechanism for change.

As is so often the case, the rhetoric hides a complex reality. Labour may not be able to accept Conservative policy in public but in private it does and agrees with Stephen Dorrell's 1996 White Paper prognosis on the future demand pressures: demography, technology and expectations are likely to be containable. No radical demand side change is therefore needed. The supply side is the place for reform. This, as I shall argue in Chapter 6, is just pushing the hardest but most real questions about health away. The evidence won't disappear, we need to ask if we spend enough on health.

Labour's main changes include creating longer term relationships between demand and supply sides of the system (purchasers and providers), stripping out costs of bureaucracy to pay for care and replacing GP fundholding with powerful primary care-based commissioning groups. But it has indicated that it will keep the purchaser/provider split.[20] However, the rhetoric and detail of its policy belies this concession. Its determination to create commissioning groups and bring in longer term relationships between purchasers and providers tends towards fudging the lines of accountability and the sharp incentives that the reformed system highlighted, replacing it with the snugness that underpinned the inefficient NHS of old. For Labour, the key challenges involve creating a less isolated and segmented hospital sector and tackling the hospital driven culture of the system – which pushes costs higher and higher – by emphasizing the status and role of primary care. Idealogically and practically, Labour's 'New NHS' is a continuation of market evolution and Conservative policy.

Chapter 3 looks at the issue of the market. It argues that the failure of market reform has meant that serious problems – outlined in the following chapters – have remained unsolved. Paradoxically, the Government must pick up on the one success of the reform – the purchaser/ provider split – to make good the real failures.

Chapter 4 looks at the issue of medical autonomy, arguing that the present series of reforms has done little to bring any accountability into the system. The market promised to deliver accountability through choice – by the patient and the purchaser. But there has been little choice. At the core of the dilemma lies the relationship between the doctor and the patient and the doctrine of clinical freedom that has allowed doctors to argue that they must place the interests of the individual patient above those of the taxpayer. Following on from this, Chapter 5 looks at the chequered history of patient and public influence over the system, suggesting that the public has never effectively been involved in the NHS. Recent reforms have emphasized chimerical patient choice over patient voice, silencing public comment to enable radical measures to be pushed through. This needs urgent redress.

Chapter 6 looks at the funding issue, arguing that it is difficult to know whether the service is underfunded, because the question – a demand-side issue – has been avoided in favour of a more politically sustainable supply-side set of reforms. There are radical proposals for changing the structures of finance using insurance systems. One key problem is that the systems do not recognize the information imbalance of the doctor–patient relationship. But there are interesting proposals that deserve appraisal.

Chapter 7 looks at the hospital network, arguing that it is inflexible, that change is needed to make it more responsive, efficient and fair, as well as maintaining quality, and that the sooner the Government devises a saleable strategy on hospital reconfiguration sensitive to local conditions the better. Closures are always resisted, and the Conservatives' problems on major hospital closures reflect their problems of confidence with the market. Labour can and must devise a successful strategy for managing reconfiguration.

Chapter 8 examines issues of medical effectiveness and quality. More needs to be done to incorporate scientifically researched medical practice into the health system – indeed the call for 'evidence based medicine' lies at the heart of Cochrane's appeal for a 'rational national health service'. Here we return to professional issues, arguing that training and traditional roles are in need of overhaul.

Chapter 9 analyses the issue of rationing, arguing that the NHS is a rationing system, stressing the need for more openness and suggesting several strategies for a national 'coming out' on the issue. Rationing is a can of worms widely predicted to be opened by the reforms. This prediction was only partially correct because of the limitations of the market.

References

1 For a review of possible future technology see (1994) The Future of Medicine. *The Economist*. **March**: 1–18. On the issues posed by advances in genetics see Macintyre S (1996) Advances in genetics: implications for health services and social and ethical issues, in M Peckham and R Smith (eds) *Scientific Basis of Health Services*. BMJ Publishing Group, London.

2 The possibilities for ever increasing care in the home are outlined in Warner M and Riley C (1994) *Closer to Home: healthcare in the 21st century*. NAHAT, Birmingham.

3 For a detailed discussion of issues of size, location and capacity of hospitals see Harrison A and Prentice S (1996) *Acute Futures*. King's Fund, London.

4 Darkins A and Sibson L (1996) *The Building of Appropriateness*. London Monitor, London.

5 Darkins A, Dearden CH, Rocke LG *et al.* (1996) An evaluation of telemedical support for a minor treatment centre. *J Telemed and Telecare*. **2**: 2.

6 Hope J (1996) The light of life. *Daily Mail*. April 2.

7 Rogers L (1996) Electric heart amazes with bodily repairs. *Sunday Times*. 10 March.

8 Leader (1996) Mr Hoffman's magic tablet. *Daily Telegraph*. 17 April.

9 For discussions of consumerism and health care see Ranade W (1994) *A Future for the NHS?* Longman, Harlow, pp. 24–46, 100–20; Spiers J (1995) *The Invisible Hospital and the Secret Garden: an insider's commentary on the NHS reforms*. Radcliffe Medical Press, Oxford, pp. xxi–xliv, 1–45; Evans R and Robinson J (1996) The role of the consumer in health research, in M Peckham and R Smith (eds) *Scientific Basis of Health Services*. BMJ Publishing Group, London.

10 DoH (1991) *The Health of the Nation: a consultative document for health in England* (Cmnd 1523). HMSO, London; DoH (1992) *The Health of the Nation* (Cmnd 1986). HMSO, London.

11 Healthcare 2000 (1995) *UK Health and Healthcare Services: challenges and policy options*. Healthcare 2000, London; Ham C and Appleby J (1995) *Background paper to the Healthcare 2000 report*. HSMC, University of Birmingham, Birmingham.

12 Laing & Buisson (1996) *Care of Elderly People: market survey*. (9th ed.) Laing & Buisson Publications, London.

13 DoH (1996) *The National Health Service: a service with ambitions* (Cmnd 3425). HMSO, London.
14 Wordsworth S, Donaldson C and Scott A (1996) *Can We Afford the NHS?* Institute of Public Policy Research, London.
15 Interview with Sir Duncan Nichol, October 1996.
16 Dr Sandy Macara, speech to BMA conference in June 1996; Dr Sandy Macara, speech to BMA conference in June 1997.
17 OECD (1996) *Health Data*. OECD, Paris.
18 For a good overview see Appleby J (1992) *Financing Healthcare in the 1990s*. Open University Press, Buckingham.
19 Bevan A (1952) *In Place of Fear*. Heinemann, London.

2 The five ages of health care

The development of medicine and the medical profession has had as much to do with the willingness of patients to believe in the power of doctors to cure them as it has with the ability of doctors to do so. At its most basic the relationship between the patient and the doctor is one of fear and hope on the one hand and almost miraculous power on the other.

From the sixteenth to the nineteenth centuries, the profession sought to institutionalize this power, and in 1948, with the creation of the NHS, it saw it nationalized.

Although the institutionalization and nationalization of medicine since the sixteenth century have been great achievements for the medical profession, they are of arguable value to today's patients and the population. Now, more than ever, there is a need for rational thinking in health care to make the system we have effective and affordable. But still public, patients and doctors relate through the traditional modes of deference and belief in the power of medicine. We do not have a rational national system.

Two key threads underpin the development of medicine and the medical profession. The first, identified by the epidemiologist Thomas McKeown suggests that historically significant improvements in health have had less to do with medicine than with urban and environmental planning.[1] The second, identified by Archie Cochrane in his 1972 Rock Carling lecture, claims that much medicine is itself ineffective and that this ineffectiveness is reinforced by the training and research practices of the profession, themselves built up over centuries of tradition and professional self-determination.[2]

These two factors combined mean the British health system may be using the wrong strategy – a medical one – to solve the problem of creating better health, which is its goal. This can be very costly, because medicine is very expensive, and will become more so.

Cultural change is coming – both to the treatment of public health and to staffing and research. But McKeown's and Cochrane's critiques of the NHS remain valuable, indicating that centuries of tradition are still locking the system into often inefficient, ineffective and inequitable practices. The success of the medical profession as a lobbying organization – through the Royal Colleges and the British Medical Association – means that alternatives to medicine – public health, environmental action – which are often cheaper, are treated as marginal, rather than core, issues by decision makers. Resolving these questions without alienating doctors – and consequently alienating a public which still sees the fight against illness as one for which only doctors are equipped – has traditionally been beyond risk-averse politicians but it is the key challenge for the NHS in the next 50 years. This chapter attempts to show how medical power has been built up.

It argues there have been five stages of medicine since the sixteenth century. In the beginning there was no effective health care. Then came a period of palliative medicine through the seventeenth and eighteenth centuries, followed by the preventative care of the nineteenth century public health movement. By the twentieth century science was giving doctors answers and the era of curative medicine dawned. The doctor was elevated in society. Finally, medicine has developed further to an ameliorative stage, where the limits of the curative model are becoming clearer. The medical profession has developed alongside it, from quackery to pillar of the British establishment.

The palliative era

If you had seen a procession of physicians walking past you some 500 years ago, you might have referred to them collectively as a 'Mystery' of doctors.[3] The early collective noun illustrates a world where doctors were perceived to possess special knowledge and were held in awe by patients. The patients, for their part, were ignorant, often fearful, forced into supplication and trust. That the doctor's repertoire was often ineffective and largely based on guesswork was beside the point. It was the belief that they could help the ill that counted.

Medicine and surgery today are often described as much as art as they are science. Their origins in medieval times, however, have as much to do with faith, religion and wizardry as they do with either. The church sought control over a profession that began to rival its own in influence: surgeons were required to pray before operations. And as the profession developed so it echoed the priesthood in setting strict entry requirements and settling itself within exclusive institutions shrouded with the rarified airs of mystery and belief.

Some key dates in the formation of the medical profession are:

• 1512 – bishops were given power to license doctors

• 1514 – licensed surgeons in London

- 1518 – Royal College of Physicians (RCP) founded in London with 12 members
- 1634 – 150 licensed apothecaries
- 1663 – RCP: 40 members
- 1600 – plague ravages Britain, medicine powerless. Advances in medicine: Harvey on circulation, Sydenham on epidemiology, Boyle in chemistry – but not applied
- 1842 – not much has changed – Byron dies of excess bleeding in company of doctors.

In the seventeenth century the status of the three groups of doctors – physicians, surgeons and apothecaries, the forerunners of GPs – was different from today. Physicians were superior, surgeons were seen as potentially murderous – their associations were not separated from the barbers until 1745. And society's view of apothecaries – only distinguished from the grocers in 1617 – is best summed up by Shakespeare's Romeo who addresses one, saying: 'Famine is in thy cheeks, need and oppression starveth in thy eyes, contempt and beggary hangs upon thy back, the world is not they friend, nor the world's law.[4] The demarcation of skills between the three was jealously guarded and there were continual disputes over who did what.

This, however, is not to say that physicians were held in high esteem. Illness was caused by an imbalance in the body's four 'humours'; the physician's job was largely to identify what was out of kilter and then bleed the patient either by cutting into a vein or applying leeches. For their part surgeons had no anaesthetic or antiseptic, and had a limited repertoire of operations including cutting holes in the skull, amputation and fixing broken bones.

This range of techniques was found wanting. Doctors did not make the connection between the bubonic plague and the rats that carried the infected fleas. Society's most prominent figures – like the philosopher Thomas Hobbes – despised doctors.[5]

Throughout the seventeenth and eighteenth centuries medical science advanced little. Mental health was neglected entirely. It was not until the twentieth century that science would begin to play a major part in medical treatments.

Preventative health

The nineteenth century was the great era of preventative health care, spurred by the Victorian public health movement led by men like the reformers Edwin Chadwick and John Simon. Chadwick believed in the fundamental importance of health – for society to function at its best it needed to have healthy citizens. Disease was wasteful: it cost money, made sufferers unproductive, and threatened the productivity of those who were well. Poor water supplies were identified as the prime causes of disease and reformers set about measures to tackle this and other threats to health. Chadwick's work is seen by many as the most important factor in improving the health of British people.[6]

The public health movement went a long way in establishing the importance of health to a successful and properly functioning modern society but the medical profession was busy too. The nineteenth century was a period of institutionalization and the foremost medical institution was the hospital.

In the seventeenth and eighteenth centuries hospitals were mainly seen as places located on the edge of towns where the poor sick were gathered together so as not to infect the rest of the population. It was in the nineteenth century that the hospitals became accepted as important institutions for the treatment of illness. They were to become the profession's power base and they provided the backdrop for a conflict that was to forge the modern medical profession and system of referral.

Key dates in the institutionalization of medicine are:

- end of 1600s – only St Thomas's and St Bartholomew's hospitals in London, few elsewhere; most rely on almshouses

- 1719–1756 – four hospitals founded

- 1770 – first public dispensary, Aldersgate, London

- 1800 – total 3000 hospital beds in Britain

- 1850s – cottage hospitals appear

- 1861 – 11 000 hospital beds.

The patchwork of hospitals that the National Health Service would inherit in 1948 was largely created by Victorian social reformers and philanthropists. It grew up around two models: the great voluntary hospitals endowed with funds by wealthy families, and the public hospitals that emerged from the workhouses established under the Poor Law for the poverty stricken and indigent.[7]

Voluntary hospitals tended to bar patients with infectious diseases or venereal disease. The workhouses grew into the public hospitals, funded with public Poor Law money, controlled by boards of guardians and were means tested.

Out of the Poor Law hospitals grew infirmaries, with more staff and a new and stronger administrative structure. Medical science advanced and doctors in voluntary hospitals began to seek only interesting, acutely ill patients, shunning the infectious or chronically sick. These were tended for in the Poor Law institutions, which became overcrowded and lacked sanitation. In addition, special hospitals were founded around particular disciplines – obstetrics, ophthalmics, paediatrics. They were set up for a number of reasons but they were often initiated by doctors who had not been accepted on to the staff of an existing voluntary hospital.

From the 1850s cottage hospitals also sprang up in rural areas not served by the major institutions. They extended the principle of payment for treatment and they permitted general practitioners into the hospitals, allowing them to perform operations on patients and to receive payment for them.

The profession was developing: the British Medical Association, known initially as the Provincial Medical and Surgical Association, was founded in 1832, and the traditional tripartite boundaries were shifting. While physicians maintained their lofty independence, the surgeons and apothecaries often became closer, particularly in the countryside. The union was the creation of the twentieth-century GP who, in the first part of the century, not only carried out tasks as family doctor but also performed operations on patients in the nearby cottage hospital. Hospital general practice was not, however, limited to the countryside. Increasingly GPs were used in the public hospitals, which lost status over time relative to the voluntary institutions.

This was a time of professional war, echoing earlier disputes between physicians and apothecaries. As GPs gained more authority, a struggle for power emerged with the consultants – physicians and surgeons in the great hospitals – who launched attacks on their innovating inferiors, who in turn accused them of 'stealing' patients.

Fees became a defining factor between the elements of the profession. The *British Medical Journal* offered them as the crucial distinction between a consultant and a GP, arguing that consultants were of superior 'culture'; had superior knowledge and so deserved superior remuneration.

The conflict created the modern system of referral which sought to formalize the transfer of patients from a private GP to a consultant – either surgeon or apothecary. The battle was bitter because the profession was fighting over the powerbase that it would occupy for the next 100 years.

This was also the period when the clinical freedom of doctors to treat patients as they saw fit, having regard solely for the welfare of the individual, casting all other considerations – including financial constraints – aside was established. It was the transition point for doctors from 'quacks' to members of society held in high regard and esteem.

Doctors insisted on both clinical freedom and the status of independent contractors as other professions and trades were being organized into salaried services and bureaucracies. As former Health Minister and doctor, David Owen, says: 'The profession was able, therefore, to establish its independence and autonomy and to free itself from the encroachment of monopoly power and bureaucracy so evident elsewhere in society, because it was able to persuade the public that medicine could be isolated from economic pressures.'[8] It led to what Owen called the 'golden age' of the medical profession, at the start of this century. But it laid the foundation for great economic and financial problems a century later.

Clinical freedom was backed up by methods of teaching that allowed the profession to regulate who joined the ranks of medicine and what treatments they would administer under the remit of clinical freedom. The training of new doctors was the key.

This principle was recognized by the monopolistic Royal Colleges in the sixteenth century and it was reaffirmed in the recruitment and training of doctors in the hospitals of the eighteenth and nineteenth centuries. The apprenticeship-based training system that hospital doctors recognize today became the method of entry and advancement in the profession. The medical profession ensured it maintained control over the process of recruitment to its ranks and training, using the hospitals as the location, underlining their function as a power base.

By the end of the nineteenth century the medical profession had established itself as an autonomous body. But one person's autonomy is another's unaccountability, and this establishment would have serious consequences for doctors, administrators, politicians and taxpayers until the present day. This autonomy preserved traditional methods of training doctors and the methods of treatment learned at medical school – many of which, to use the current jargon, are not 'evidence based'. The tradition of passing treatments from one generation to the next has resulted in many being incorporated into the body of medical practice for no other reason than that they were done before, and are 'tried and tested'.

Other principles that were established at this time were the blurring of the distinction between private practice and free medicine – the use of early 'pay beds' and the right of doctors to treat patients in voluntary hospitals like Guy's is an example – an issue that has remained a running controversy to the present day. Again, the independent contractor status on which doctors insisted in the nineteenth century has remained a constant source of negotiation and argument ever since.

As the hospitals grew, so did the administrative side, with governors appointing secretaries and clerks. The development of a bipartite structure based around a house committee and a medical committee, with the house committee having the final word in disputes, created a tension that has remained through the managerial reforms of the present-day health system – both public and private.

As seeds of controversy were sown, however, so were those of great future benefit. As we have seen, the referral process between GPs and consultants was established at this time. That, as Iona Heath has observed, had beneficial long-term consequences: 'This fortuitous outcome has been one of the great successes of the British health care system and the foundation of its widely recognised cost effectiveness.'[3]

So, at the close of the nineteenth century, the medical profession had established itself as a pillar of the new middle classes, controlling entry, practice, remuneration, terms and conditions of work, and commanding unprecedented public respect. All this despite the fact that it was those involved in public health who were and are credited with having made the greatest advances in health during the period.

The philanthropic Victorian model of health care was unsustainable, however, and as it declined, so a new system grew up to take its place – the Welfare State. Britain's welfare system was founded by David Lloyd George in 1911, on the principles of insurance. Benefits of the scheme were dependent on the contributions made to it. It was a system that would later be scrapped when the National Health Service was created and paid for out of general tax revenues but it lasted in roughly the form in which it had been created in 1911 until the Second World War.

The creation of the Welfare State made a strong impact on the medical profession. Doctors were determined not to surrender determination of their methods or conditions of work or payment for it to outsiders – particularly the Government. The introduction of the Lloyd George system was, as the introduction of the National Health Service would be some 37 years later, fiercely resisted by the doctors. They feared becoming direct employees of the State, and negotiated payment per patient on their list rather than by receiving a salary as well as making participation in the insured 'panel' scheme optional, not compulsory. They were also able to negotiate generous fees, and exclude the wealthy – who still paid their own way from the panel system along with the families of insured people. Nevertheless, after the Second World War the scheme incorporated two thirds of GPs and included 21 million people – though only workers, not their families, were covered.

With the foundation of the Welfare State came another profound change in the profession: the politicization of medicine. As the State took greater responsibility for financing, so medicine and politics became ever more closely linked until, with the creation of the National Health Service in 1948, the two were inextricably bound together. At the same time health care moved into its fourth phase: the curative.

Curative medicine

Two significant developments characterized health care in the twentieth-century. The first was the ascendancy of high technology medicine and the doctor and the second was the nationalization and politicization of health care. A series of medical breakthroughs including the discovery of sulphonamide antibiotics and penicillin allied to improvements in anaesthetics increased the status of the modern doctor and lent weight to the claims of medicine to be a scientific process that could be proven to benefit patients and improve health. Whether or not these developments were the fundamental causes of the increased well-being of British people has, as we have seen, been questioned.[1] What was indisputable, however, was that the establishment of hospitals around the country had made medicine more widely available. Coupled to the development of the medical profession during the public health era, these advances helped to establish a 'medical model' of health based around cure and medical intervention by doctors, over and above prevention of the causes of ill health by wider society. This allowed medical dominance of the nationalization and politicization of health care in the NHS.

As Chris Ham points out:

> Acceptance of the medical model is important, first, in justifying the pre-eminent position of the medical profession in health matters and second, in helping to explain the pattern of investment in health services. Within the NHS, the bulk of resources is allocated to personally orientated, general and acute hospital services. Much less importance has been attached to collective, preventative and welfare approaches to health.[10]

The medical model dictated these spending patterns up to and beyond the foundation of the National Health Service. More money has traditionally been spent on building, staffing and financing hospitals than was ever spent on community or preventative services.

Indeed, throughout the negotiations that led to the foundation of the National Health Service one thing became clear: it would in fact operate as a National Medical Service. And this was a view the medical profession went out of its way to promote.

The underlying message of the medical profession's campaigns – not least of which was the popular lobbying television programme *Your Life in Their Hands* – was to show itself at the cutting edge of technology, to emphasize its competence and its right to clinical freedom on the one hand and a say in how the system was set up and administered on the other.

It was during war that the template for the NHS was set up from the foundations of the wartime Emergency Hospital Service, which brought all hospitals under national control to deal with casualties.[11] As Rudolf Klein points out, the system was hopelessly complicated and needed to be sorted out. It was a spirit of rationalism that prompted the inter-war reformers to think of ways of reforming what was a very muddled system. The scientific rationalism that allowed doctors to find cures for previously intractable diseases, it was thought, ought to be transferred to social science, allowing health care, if not health, to be distributed evenly across the country.[11]

The question of payment remained high on the doctors' agenda. Allied to the issue of payment was that of private practice, a problem that would absorb Bevan in his attempts to get the doctors to accept his system some ten years later. The BMA stated that voluntary hospitals were no longer strictly charitable and the majority of patients treated there could and did pay. It argued that doctors should be able to charge patients who could afford to pay to maintain their own standards of living.

The definition of what constituted a consultant was sharpened. Control of the membership of the profession was still a matter of the utmost importance. According to the BMA, consultants, therefore, held or had held hospital appointments, where they had acquired 'special skill and experience of the kind required for the performance of the service rendered', had studied at postgraduate level, and were 'generally recognised by other practitioners in the area as having special proficiency and experience in a subject which comprises the service rendered.' The relationship between consultants and GPs was once again laid out, re-opening the disputes that had occupied the profession for so long.

In 1944 a White Paper was published, arguing for a comprehensive and free national health service. The report's author, Henry Willink made a number of concessions to the BMA on grievances that were, by then, well recognized. General practitioners were to be given the choice of salaried payment or capitation fees. Doctors' contracts were to be negotiated between the Government and the BMA, and a Central Medical Board was to oversee the distribution of doctors over the country, though it could not, as in previous plans, prevent doctors from selling their premises. Local Government would have responsibility for primary and community care, joint authorities would control the municipal hospitals and the service would be financed by National Insurance.

But the plan upset the doctors. They were suspicious of a salaried service and did not like the involvement of the local authorities or the idea of the service being comprehensive, fearing this would undermine private practice. In a postal poll, the doctors came out strongly against the plan.

But there was great public support for a free NHS. When Sir William Beveridge's 1942 report had stated that alongside universal child allowances and a policy to reduce unemployment, a free national health service for prevention and treatment of disease was to be made available to all, the public rejoiced.

The Labour Health Minister and architect of the NHS, Aneurin Bevan, combined the qualities of idealism and political skill vital to the creation of the NHS. When he arrived in Whitehall, Bevan faced a profession rendered defensive by the 1944 proposals: doctors feared losing their independent contractor status, becoming in effect civil servants in the new nationalized service. Bevan proposed to take the hospitals into State control, as had been suggested by a senior civil servant, Arthur McNalty, in 1940. To do this he needed to wrest them from those institutions that controlled them, placing them under the administrative control of regional hospital boards and district committees. This caused confrontation with both local government – which controlled the municipal hospitals – and the medical profession, which still guarded its control of the voluntary ones.

In return for enlisting the salaried services of specialists in the NHS, Bevan gave the teaching hospitals – the voluntary organizations by now run by consultants – self-governing status with their own boards. He also allowed doctors to sit on the new regional health boards and enshrined in the NHS legislation the right of consultants to work in private practice. This effectively ensured a second, higher stream of income, for doctors in addition to the security of the NHS. It also created a private sector that evolved alongside the NHS. The insurance-based system of paying for private care that has existed since then, was set up under the eye of the medical profession, keen to ensure people could pay for private treatment when they needed it. The health insurance movement received a new invigoration from the foundation of the NHS – the British United Provident Association dates from 1947. Lastly Bevan accepted proposals for a system of merit awards by which specialists are given payment over and above their salaries as a reward for service and good practice. The payments were awarded by doctors.

When questioned some years later as to how he had managed to get the service off the ground with the consultants on board, Bevan replied famously 'I stuffed their mouths with gold.'

Bevan also had to deal with the GPs, suspicious of being left with the fag end of the NHS deal. He made a concession by retaining the insurance committees that had administered the panel system. This maintained the independent contracting status of the GPs.

Proposals for remuneration – on a mixture of salary and capitation – and for the new Medical Practices Committee to oversee where practices were set up and ensuring equal distribution throughout the country, did not go down so well. The GPs, urged on by the BMA, threatened not to join the service until weeks before it started in 1948. It was only through dropping the salaried element of payment that Bevan managed to get them on board.

Through a mixture of compromise and cajoling, then, Bevan managed to get the NHS off the ground on 5 July 1948. A tripartite system was set up in 1948 – the hospital service run by regional hospital boards and teaching hospital boards of governors, accountable to central government; community services provided by local government through social services committees; and primary care administered by separate executive councils, which could trace their ancestry back to the pre-war insurance committees. It was intended to bring the best medical treatment to all, whereas before it had only been available in areas where it could be paid for – generally by those least in need of it. The new scheme saw consultants spreading into the countryside instead of being concentrated in the affluent areas of the south east.

From the outset the tripartite structure thrashed out in the compromise between Bevan and the medical profession undermined efficiency and equity within the system. There was also the problem of expanding demand.

The question of funding and efficiency prompted an enquiry into NHS financing, chaired by Claude Guillebaud, a Cambridge economist and former tutor of the then Health Minister Ian Macleod. The Committee of Enquiry into the Cost of the National Health Service, as it was called, was charged with discovering why, when the Government actuary had stated that the NHS would cost about £170 million a year to run Bevan had had to announce a revision upwards to £225 million within only four months.[12,13]

From the early days two pressures worked on the NHS to produce a series of reforms to its structure: the need to spread the service and to rationalize its administration.

Drawn up under Enoch Powell, the 1962 Hospital plan looked to do something Bevan had never found time to do: updating the hotchpotch of 2800 voluntary and municipal hospitals, half of which dated back to before 1891. The country was analysed, region by region, to assess the need for new hospitals. The chaotic system of small hospitals was to be rationalized into a network of large, modern units, where technology would bring down lengths of stay, and therefore costs. In addition, the steep regional variations in provision were to be narrowed. Along with the spread of technology, came the spread of the medical powerbase.[14]

Another change was the reorganization of the health service in 1974, prepared by Keith Joseph during the Heath government and brought in by Barbara Castle after Harold Wilson won the election of that year.

The reorganization was aimed at unifying the tripartite service. But the unification was unsuccessful. General practitioners maintained their autonomy by keeping executive committees out of reach of health authorities and retaining direct funding from departments. The merger finally occurred in 1996 when the committees' descendants, family health service authorities, were merged with health authorities. It was intended to boost the Cinderella services – mental health and community care – shifting them away from local authorities to health authorities.[15] This too was a damp squib. It was also intended to improve co-ordination – for example by making area health authorities cover the same areas as local authorities, creating joint consultative committees to co-ordinate the different authorities. The third aim was to improve management through multi-disciplinary team working, consensus management and drawing in doctors to the management function.

The success of these changes was limited: the service neither became unified nor desperately communicative, and the consensus management system became seen as responsible for many of the NHS's ills, particularly its inability to curb the costs of expensive high tech. medicine. What it did indicate, however, was that perceptions of the limitations of management coloured all thinking about how the NHS should be reformed.

Ameliorative care

The 1974 reorganization grappled with important problems in the health service – a chaotic hospital system and fragmented management. But it did not deal with the latent tensions that had existed since before the foundation of the post-war health system and which became more visible as time wore on. These tensions gradually resolved themselves into two pressing questions for which there had to be wider political, rather than narrowly NHS-based, answers. The first was how to make up a widening gap between demand for services and the ability to pay for them. The second was whether the medical settlement, based on the consensus between doctor, administrator, politician and taxpayer was sustainable.

Simply stated, a new dilemma faced the NHS. Economic growth was slowing and so, to keep public services at historical levels – essential politics – public spending grew as a proportion of GDP. At the same time public willingness to pay taxes for services they perceived to be in decline instead of keeping the money to spend as they thought best was being tested. People were unwilling to spend more of their total wealth in taxes on services while the services needed more of the national cake to run at the levels at which people had become accustomed. Something would have to give.

At the same time, medicine entered the latest phase: the ameliorative phase. The scientific exuberance of the post-war era began to subside with the realization that many chronic conditions – cardio-vascular diseases, respiratory conditions, cancers – had to be managed, often expensively, because they could not be cured. Some contagious diseases reappeared – in Britain, for example, the number of people under 70 dying from TB increased in 1990/91 for the first time after decades of decline.[16] The growth of counselling and alternative therapies, and even the reintroduction of leeches, all suggested that a view of health care beyond traditional medicine was growing.

The view now is that medicine may be able to save your life, but you will have to bear the consequences of treatment, which can take a heavy toll. Medicine, in other words, is a trade-off between treatment and lifestyle and the results are often at best ameliorative. The 1970s saw the beginnings of attempts by economists to quantify this – to help with setting priorities in health care.

The accountability issue was fundamental. The medical profession had largely succeeded in maintaining its autonomy through its negotiations with Bevan, and this was not substantially altered until the 1980s, despite sometimes ferocious confrontations with different governments. The pressures that flowed from this – the separation of treatment from its financial consequences, the effectiveness of treatment, the methods of recruitment and training – were all maintained, but doctors, so dominant in the formation of the NHS, soon found that reformers were less willing to listen and, indeed, were even hostile to them.

As money grew scarcer and medicine's power was ever more widely questioned, the hidden mechanics of the system operated less smoothly. The problem of managing exploding demand presented itself. The issue of rationing became ever more prominent and changed in character from the accepted process of the post-war days. The question of equity went hand-in-hand with this. Balanced against it was the problem of extracting greater efficiency. The issue of centralization or devolution of power became pressing. The balance of power between consultants and GPs, and between both and health service administrators, was problematic.

In short, the post-war consensus was preserved until the Conservative Government in the 1980s judged that it posed too great a burden on public funds for management by the effectively self-regulated medical profession to be allowed to continue. However, the Government, never able to reject the underlying principles of the NHS, could only alter the consensus without being able to blast it away.

Attempts at reform were restricted to the supply side. In order to rein in expenditure on the service a link had to be forged between decisions made on clinical grounds and their economic consequences. This meant challenging the historic clinical freedom of the medical profession. It was here that the first of the two major changes brought about by the 1980s Conservative governments was aimed. In 1983–84 an enquiry into the management of the NHS, led by Sainsbury's managing director Roy Griffiths, led to the introduction of general management, to forge a link between the world of medicine and the world of budgets – in short, to create financial accountability.[17]

The latest reforms introduced in the National Health Service and Community Care Act of 1990 dismissed altering the funding of the service, and again concentrated on reforming the supply side. They created an 'internal market' in the NHS in a series of measures.[18]

The first was that purchasers and providers of health care were to be separated. Before 1990, district health authorities had been allocated funds by central government and used them to run their local hospitals. After 1990 the hospital role was taken away from the authorities and they were left as purchasers, with a duty to assess the health needs of their local populations and purchase services for them. To do this they entered into contracts with newly formed hospital trusts, which were introduced in five waves as the reforms were gradually implemented over the country. The intention was to allow purchasers to move contracts between providers to provoke competition between them. In placing contracts with providers for a type and volume of service, the reforms intended to make 'money follow the patient'. The third element of the reforms was the GP fundholder. The introduction of GP fundholding along with purchasing was intended to reverse the pre-eminence of consultants and 'producers' of health care. General practitioners and health authorities took responsibility for quality for their patients and sought value for the taxpayer.

Underneath the disparate elements of reform was the attempt – often unsuccessful – to make the system more rational. A rational NHS was the dream of many, but the means of achieving it were never more clearly articulated than by Archie Cochrane in the 1970s. He believed the system was inefficient and poorly managed, unaccountable and unjust. And the reason for this, he believed, was the medical establishment itself. Far from being a triumph of scientific rationalism, the service embodied the unscientific methods of a medical priesthood unwilling to loosen its grip on power. Management inefficiency and ineffectiveness, he believed, all flowed from this central problem.[2]

The role of the doctor and the relationship with the patient has undergone some fundamental change since the sixteenth century. For some people, however, the medical profession maintains its mystery, and the public retains its awe. John Spiers, formerly chief executive of a large trust hospital, says: 'Public solace in medicine is often sought where it is embedded culturally – in myth and mystique.[19]

As well as rationalizing pressure that had been hidden within the system before, and attempting to introduce a notion of efficiency, the reforms are also fundamentally redefining the relationships between the key players in the health arena. Before the latest reforms, changes in policy adjusted pressures and altered the balance of power between the dominant medical profession and politicians, administrators and patients. Now, however, a new set of relationships is taking shape.

Key among these is the consumer. If the power of producers was to be broken – and this was one of the key commandments of Conservative reform in the 1980s – the power of the consumer looking for choice and value, with the market as a tool for doing so, was the method. Here we return to the beginning of this chapter, to the relationship between doctor and patient, to the almost mysterious link between the two based on history, fear and uncertainty. This belief is what Margaret Thatcher set out to break with the management reforms of the 1980s and, when she saw these had not worked properly she set out to smash it with the health reforms of the 1990s. But she and her successors never took the issue head on, never attempted to open up the mysterious duality that underpins modern medicine.

The reforms were intended to bring decisions on spending taxpayers' money as close to the consumer of health services as possible using the proxy of the health authority or, preferably, the fundholding GP to choose between providers on cost and quality, thus enhancing efficiency. At all times information is the key, and price the guide.

Alongside the elevation of the consumer has been the elevation of the administrator, acting as the consumer's proxy – although recent policy has been to play down the importance of managers. Beginning with the Griffiths Report, the administrator was converted into a manager. Instead of complying with the medical profession, he was required to assess its performance and instil in it the notion of value for money.

But the idea of 'letting the market rip' was never carried out in practice in the way it was intended, and it has faded further into the background of the health agenda. The market is now being played down.

The question of the place of doctors within the health system and wider society really comes down to that of what we want them to be. As patients we want them to do the best for us. As taxpayers we want them to be efficient. But we can't have a cheap service when we don't need it and an expensive one when we do. A notion of wider responsibility has to become rooted in the patient if it is to be a part of the medical practice. Once we are clear about this we can start setting boundaries for what we expect the system to achieve, boundaries that are visible, fair, and that make it clear to us before we use the system how much we can expect out of it. It is difficult for doctors to say to patients they cannot afford treatments when those patients expect care to be free and comprehensive. If patients were made aware that rationing has always existed, but that to make it fairer it must become clearer, then a more rational debate could start.

It remains to be seen if consumers empowered with information and knowledge can challenge the self-importance, mystery and mystique of the medical profession and whether they feel it is right for them to do so. It remains to be seen whether people want to take responsibility. It could be that we have travelled far since the sixteenth century, only to find we have moved nowhere when we sit in the doctor's chair and begin to open our hearts, glad to be able to switch off our minds.

References

1 McKeown T (1976) *The Modern Rise of Population and the Role of Medicine: dream, mirage or nemesis?* Nuffield Provincial Hospitals Trust, London.
2 Cochrane A (1971) *Effectiveness and Efficiency: random reflections on health services.* Nuffield Provincial Hospitals Trust, London.
3 Heath I (1995) *The Mystery of General Practice.* John Fry Trust Fellowship, Nuffield Provincial Hospitals Trust, London.
4 William Shakespeare. *Romeo and Juliet,* Act V, scene I.
5 For some fascinating examples of how medicine was wrapped-up with belief systems see Thomas K (1971) *Religion and the Decline of Magic.* Weidenfeld & Nicolson, London, pp. 3–24, 98–100, 308–10, 328–9, 512–14, 640–1.
6 Finer SE (1952) *The Life and Times of Sir Edwin Chadwick.* Methuen, London.
7 For a historical analysis of British hospitals see Abel-Smith B (1964) *The Hospitals 1800–1948.* Heinemann, London; Ham C (1992) *Health Policy in Britain.* (3rd ed.) Macmillan, Basingstoke.
8 Owen D (1988) *Our NHS.* Pan Books, London.
9 Ham C (1992) *Op Cit.*; Honigsbaum F (1989) *Health, Happiness and Security: the creation of the National Health Service.* Routledge, London.
10 Ham C (1992) *Op Cit.* p. 225.
11 For historical background on the foundation of the modern health system see Timmins N (1995) *The Five Giants: a biography of the welfare state.* HarperCollins, London; Klein R (1995) *The New Politics of the National Health Service.* (3rd ed.) Longman, Harlow.

12 Bevan A (1952) *In Place of Fear*. Heinemann, London.
13 Guillebaud C (1956) *Report of the Committee of Enquiry into the National Health Service* (Cmnd 9663). HMSO, London.
14 Minister of Health (1962) *A Hospital Plan for England and Wales* (Cmnd 1604). HMSO, London.
15 Ham C (1992) *Op Cit.* pp. 24–30.
16 OECD (1996) *Health Data*. OECD, Paris.
17 Griffiths R (1983) *NHS Management Inquiry*. DHSS, London.
18 Secretaries of State for Health, Wales, Northern Ireland and Scotland (1989) *Working for Patients* (Cmnd 555). HMSO, London; *The National Health Service and Community Care Act 1990*. HMSO, London. A good summary of the early implementation of the reforms can be found in Ranade W (1994) *A Future for the NHS?* Longman, Harlow, pp. 46–65.
19 Spiers J (1997) *Who Owns Our Bodies? making moral choices in health care.* Radcliffe Medical Press, Oxford.

3 Market? What market?

The internal market is the single most unpopular thing in British health care. The Government has pledged to 'abolish' it. The previous Government distanced itself from it as soon as it had invented it. The medical profession is split by it in more ways than one and the public is suspicious of it. Yet there are elements of the internal market system that have proved to be of great value. If it has done anything it has taught us the value of information for analysis. It would be foolish to cast away this considerable step forward in the name of ideology.

On one level, therefore, the Government is foolish in promising to end the internal market, but if we look behind the rhetoric, the Government recognizes its value, although whether it will maintain its effectiveness is unclear. Understanding the use to which information can be put in reshaping the health system is one thing. Accepting the conclusions to which greater information points and following these conclusions through into action is, however, an entirely different question. But this is a problem facing all parties. Labour defines replacing the market as doing away with annual contracting in favour of longer term 'service agreements' and replacing GP fundholding, while keeping the purchaser/provider split – which produces pressure for open and analytical use of information in commissioning services as well as allowing purchasers to switch providers. The first measure may undermine the second.[1]

The debate over the market is streaked through with ironies. The starting point is that there is no such thing as a market in health. We cannot buy, sell, commission or provide wellness or unwellness. We can only do this for health care – and that market destroys itself. Consequently, the second point is that the market system that was introduced to gain the benefits of analysis had to be so emasculated as not to work properly at all. The question therefore presents itself – is the Government talking tough about abolishing something that never existed? The third point is that, given the Government is to keep the purchaser/provider split, is it 'abolishing' anything at all?

Why doesn't the market work?

In economic theory the relationship between the individual and medicine is too difficult for the patient to take decisions on diagnosis and treatment. Doctors are the next best thing. The information is complex, so the patient usually hands over responsibility to an 'agent' – the GP. This is an example of 'market failure', leaving open the possibility of exploitation of the consumer (patient) by the producer (doctor). The financial problem arises when payment comes into the relationship either directly by the patient or indirectly by the state or an insurance company. Normal rules of exchange do not work.[2]

One of the key problems – known as cream skimming – faced by a private system on a wide scale has been illustrated by the American experience, where before the Second World War insurance companies were set up to cover wide populations for health costs that were rising. The original companies were known as the 'Blues', because they were named Blue Cross and Blue Shield – and offered cover for large numbers of people on the understanding that they would take anyone who approached them for cover.

To start with, the Blues were successful, making reasonable returns on offering cover. However, as the market developed, other companies wanted to enter and they were more choosy about who they signed up. They concentrated on younger, fitter groups, excluding the costly elderly. At the same time they offered lower premiums than the Blues to entice the young away from the schemes. The result was that the young and healthy went to the new companies, which were successful for a time – until they themselves were undercut.

So, while the new companies were collecting premium income and not paying out, the Blues were left with the older, higher claimants, and therefore found that the money they collected in premiums was quickly eaten up again by claims. They had no wider population to spread the burden of payment because they had all left for the lower premium companies, and so their risk was concentrated.

Another problem for insurers is moral hazard. Once individuals are insured there is little incentive for them not to claim on the policy. This can happen both in private and public systems and is a key reason for rising premium costs in the one case and the increasing burden put on public finances on the other. Without control over claims both public and private systems can run into trouble. Thus private systems have emulated the American Health Maintenance Organization model, which seeks to establish control over care costs through provisions in policies. The NHS has an inbuilt claims management system in the GP gatekeeper, and one of the functions of the fundholding system was to strengthen this role. Some health authorities are using HMO models to build their own 'managed care' systems.

In addition, there are equity problems; specifically, in a market with choice there will not be equal access or use made of health services because of varying power by consumers to exercise choice: in short that those in equal need may not receive equal treatment.[3]

It was to overcome these problems – acutely felt in Britain before the Second World War that the NHS was created – to banish uncertainty, inaccessibility and unaffordability from the provision of health services for good. But that has become more and more expensive.

The answer – an internal market

The internal or 'quasi' market was introduced into the NHS to produce a politically acceptable solution to an increasingly unattractive economic reality. It had to obtain more value from the resources that were being put into the service without undermining the universal free treatment at the point of delivery that was its justification, which would have happened if a free market had been created. So it was to be managed to prevent market failure.

A 'quasi market', therefore ought to be judged by its ability to increase the efficiency and responsiveness of a service and promote choice while maintaining equity as far as possible. Resistance to the theory of the market and its search for efficiency has been strong in the NHS, but, as two authors say: 'There is nothing caring about wasting resources.'[4]

Efficiency does not mean simply that the lowest cost is the best. If a hospital is knocking out low-cost joint operations to attract fundholders and health authorities to send their patients, only to find that they need their joints replaced again five or ten years down the line, then it is not efficient. Ideas of quality must be included, so that efficiency means the lowest possible cost for an accepted quality of work.

Choice for the user of welfare services has been an alien idea, but it is the underpinning of market efficiency – purchasers must be able to choose between providers if there is to be an incentive to produce quality and good value. Choice is a more complicated notion than it appears at first and needs to be examined in the case of health services.

According to Le Grand and Bartlett: although the reforms 'are being driven by a government [the Conservatives] for which equity considerations are not necessarily a high priority', the NHS is part of a welfare state, and 'since the motivation that underlay the creation of the welfare state in the first place was in large part the promotion of greater social justice or equity, no evaluation of the success or otherwise of a particular set of welfare reforms would be complete without reference to equity criteria.'[4] As we shall see in a later chapter, the NHS performs well in terms of equity when compared with others. Some commentators believe, however, that equity has been sacrificed for the goal of increased efficiency.

The concept is a complex one, however. What do we mean by equity? One study points to five different definitions of equity: health care funding distributed equally to each person, according to financial need, according to health or sickness, in proportion to capacity to benefit, or to promote equal outcomes of health. Clarity is needed about which of these is being promoted.[5]

The market itself must have a structure allowing it to function correctly. It should be 'contestable' – there should be enough providers for purchasers to choose from, allowing them to influence price by the threat or the action of moving their business from one place to another, and to avoid monopoly. There should be choice at the entry of the system, between the GPs, for those GPs and between providers.

There should also be flexibility – new providers should have easy access to the market, and poor ones should be squeezed out. Prices themselves should reflect supply and demand and should be able to move freely, or as freely as possible when a transaction is made.

There must be adequate information allowing cost and price information to be given and quality monitoring to be carried out. It must also limit the scope of providers to take advantage of their position as holders of most information. A hospital may fail to provide the level of service agreed without the purchaser or patient being any the wiser. Contracts themselves determine the type and amount of information available and how easy it is to change circumstances.

The internal market reforms

The internal market was seen as the best way of dealing with the specific problems presented by the British health system. By 1979 the pattern of health care had been changing and economic pressures were building strongly.

- The number of inpatients had grown by more than 2% a year.

- The elderly population had grown by more than 2% a year from 1961 whereas the population as a whole grew by only 0.3% over the same period.

- There were fewer patients to each doctor.
- Technology increased costs and the specialization of work – there were some 55 specialties.
- The growth of general practice – contact rates between GPs and the population was growing rapidly.
- Spending on health had risen as a proportion of GDP from 3.9% in 1960, to 4.5% in 1970 to 5.6% in 1980.

The medical profession and clinical freedom represented a barrier to confronting these economic challenges. They were seen as a great vested interest, buttressed by the centuries old Hippocratic principle of devotion to the individual. With the foundation of the NHS there was a new imperative – a responsibility to the taxpayer and society at large. But this had never been directly addressed.

Before the days of a tax-funded system it was easier to answer the question 'to whom is the doctor accountable?' by saying simply 'the patient'. Now this had to be balanced by accountability to the taxpayer, or the taxpayer's proxy, the manager – either purchaser or provider.

The BMA made it clear that the individual patient came first.

> Within the NHS resources are finite and this may restrict the freedom of the doctor to advise his patient ... The doctor has a general duty to advise on equitable allocation and efficient utilisation (but this) is subordinate to his professional duty to the individual who seeks his clinical advice.[6]

Failure to resolve the issue of the economic impact of clinical freedom underlay many of the difficulties the system faced, but the Government was unwilling to alter the relationship explicitly, so maintaining the focus on the individual, which would allow doctors not to face the financial consequences of their actions. An alternative strategy was to make doctors accountable by creating an adversarial relationship between those in primary care and those in hospitals, and to give managers teeth. The fundamental tension in the system was not addressed and the attempt to superimpose a new culture of accountability massively increased it. Those responsible for making the hard choices – fundholding GPs and health authority and hospital managers – were vilified by hospital medical staff and non-fundholders. But as they poured derision on the new system, their targets pointed out that they absolved their critics of taking the hard choices themselves. They should have been thanked not scorned.

The Griffiths Report of 1982 introduced general managers into the NHS in an attempt to forge the link between clinicians and costs, and introduced cost improvement programmes that led to annual savings of between 1.1% and 1.5% a year after their introduction in 1986.[7]

The spirit of general management started at the top with the creation of the Health Services Supervisory Board and the NHS management board, chaired by a manager from outside the NHS. Day-to-day responsibility was devolved to unit level as far as possible, and budgets were to be set within each unit with a clearly defined financial framework. Management budgets were set up involving clinicians, and relating workload and service objectives to financial and manpower allocations to ensure easier analysis of costs. And the management of NHS property was transformed with NHS interest and depreciation charges for use of capital and the ability to borrow for projects to make sure estates were managed efficiently instead of being treated by hospitals as 'gifts' of the state. There was also to be a review of staff to reduce numbers, and an attempt to make the public more aware of what the NHS could realistically be expected to deliver.[8]

Alongside these changes came a new structure for managing hospitals. The principle was that senior doctors should take control of 'clinical directorates' usually overseeing a specialty, accountable to the hospital board through an overall medical director.

Political interference at a central level reduced the autonomy and power that managers had to make change count. Management was successful in some health authorities but not in others. At a local level, as Chris Ham points out: 'general managers have not found it easy to develop more effective working relationships with hospital doctors.' Even the general managers who welcomed the principles of the reform package were often confused as to how to go about implementing them.[9]

Within four years it was apparent that a more fundamental shift was needed. A major reason was that the Griffiths Report had not cracked medical power because it had not addressed the issue of clinical freedom. According to the American academic Alain Enthoven, who strongly influenced the Government's thinking on the market reforms that were to come 'The consultants ... have accepted long-term contracts with the NHS and limits on total expenditure in exchange for job security and "clinical freedom". Thus NHS management has very little leverage to make their services more responsive to patients' needs.'[10]

To this he added independent GPs, who were 'politically powerful and have no desire to yield their autonomy' and who had no incentive to reduce referrals to hospitals. Managers were 'afraid to rock the boat' and local MPs were in the thrall of doctors.

There were 'perverse incentives', which made it in a consultant's interest to keep his or her waiting lists up to boost their own private practice with people who wanted to jump the queue. The Griffiths Report recommendations were laudable but were unworkable in the current culture of the NHS. 'There are too many ways the doctors and staff can defeat the general manager if they don't perceive the manager's ideas to be in their interest,' Enthoven said.[10] General managers in short were unable to counter these ingrained power structures.

The failures of Griffiths were confronted in 1989, with the publication of the *Working for Patients* White Paper, which introduced three fundamental changes. First, the hitherto integrated health system would be split into a contract-based internal market, with health authority and GP purchasers buying care from hospitals, which would have to compete for contracts. Second, hospitals were to come out of health authority control to become free-standing trusts. Third, GPs could become fundholders, purchasing services with their own budgets. The budgets were split between hospital services and prescribing, both being cash limited for the first time. The market would achieve what management had failed to deliver.

The efficiency, effectiveness and value of doctors and hospitals was to be judged on commercial terms – by contracts. If you were good you would get plenty of work. If you were not, you would not. The key was the freedom of the purchaser to choose so that money flowed through the system according to the choices it made – it would follow the patient.

The system was to operate on two fronts. The first was to shift the emphasis of the service away from the hospital and into the community, where general practitioners would fulfil greater roles in possession of budgets that would forge a link between the treatment they offered and its cost. General practitioners were to become accountable for their spending on secondary care through fundholding, as well as through stronger audit procedures and tighter controls on drug budgets. They would be accountable for the quality of service for their patients and would use those patients to track the performance of the system as they went through it.

The second front was making the hospitals – the providers – accountable through contracts to the GP fundholders and health authorities – the purchasers – on the outside and stronger management within. What was planned was: 'A transition from an "implicit, unspoken concordat between the state and the medical profession", in which the former provided funds and the latter allocated them, to an explicit, contractually defined relationship between the holders of the public purse and the providers of care.'[11]

Box 3:1 Contract deadlock

David Thomas is finance director of Chase Farm Hospital in Enfield, North London. Chase Farm is a district general hospital and its main contracts are with the local purchaser, Enfield and Haringey Health Authority. In 1994/95, Chase Farm's income was £47.2 million. In 1996 the contracts between the Chase Farm and Enfield and Haringey were not agreed until the late summer after they had been through an arbitration process to force an agreement. The problems stemmed from the 3% efficiency index requirement – that Chase Farm provides either the same level of service for 3% less or 3% more for the same money. In the words of one manager: 'We have found it very difficult to deliver.'

Mr Thomas says: 'We have no regard for Enfield and Haringey's ability. We feel that despite what they said in their report to the arbitrator, they have a high regard for our ability. That may be arrogant of us, but it makes life very difficult and has made negotiations this year very difficult. They decide what services they want, at what level and what quality. Then they are supposed to come to us with the documentation; a purchasing plan and the document they produced did not add up.'

Another problem was that the health authority refused to pay for any services it considered to be 'developmental', saying it could only pay for a core of services that were needed by the population. Chase Farm argued that all their services had elements that were developmental; the nature of medicine is that it is always advancing. All their prices therefore had developmental costs built into them and if they were not going to be paid for developing services they would end up not being paid anything.

David Thomas says: 'Our contracts with Enfield and Haringey are all block. That means we take all the risk for providing services.' Say a health authority made a block contract payment to a trust for a year's services for its population, with no indication of the volume of services, under which the trust decided to budget for £1 million on hip replacements. Say each one cost £3500. If non-fundholding GPs referred less than 285 people to have hip replacements, the hospital would be able to provide the service at a surplus. If more than that were referred it would be supplied at a loss.

The hospital's view is that as contracts are negotiated with an eye to waiting lists and past volumes, health authorities are able to off-load the risk on to hospitals so that the likely referrals exceed the value of the contract. In Enfield and Haringey, fundholding GPs work on a different basis, negotiating cost and volume contracts. Here benchmarks are set on a block basis, but anything over this mark is paid for on a cost per case basis, so the hospital receives the money it spends on treating the excess.

The health authority view was that the hospital was not being efficient or reasonable in the contracting round. A spokesman for the health authority explained its side of the story, saying: 'From our perspective the main problems were the increased costs of the provider linked to a very expansionist view about the services they wanted to develop without taking into account the views of the health authority.' He said problems centred around the question of having 24 hour theatre coverage in the hospital and the need for more staff appointments – the hospital said they needed to expand midwifery services and needed a series of consultant appointments. The question was not that these extras were not desirable but whether they were necessarily the best things to be spending health authority money on. The health authority spokesman said: 'It ended up that they wanted us to fund an extra 15 midwife places and we said we could only afford an extra two. The Regional Office decided and in the end there was a compromise – we funded five.' He continued: 'The health authority's view was that it should be a decision of the health authority to decide on what to spend, rather than the trust. But I felt the trust was very aggressive. In the end, I think we were the more reasonable but I think this all goes to show that the contracting system does not necessarily work very well. I think there should be greater co-operation between trusts and health authorities, moving to longer periods of contracting – these annual rows may then be easier in the long term.'

Interviews with David Thomas, July/September 1996 and Enfield and Haringey Health Authority, December 1996.

Why doesn't the internal market work?

Many of the problems of the internal market come through attempts to limit the logic of the real market.

Information, choice and the individual

Choice was intended as the fulcrum of each relationship in the reformed system. It allowed the patient to choose fundholders, who would try and attract patients because they came with funds. It allowed the fundholder to choose the best treatment on behalf of the patient. The importance of choice reflects two strands in thinking about patients and individuals: first that they are capable of making decisions about health care, and second that bringing choice based on information on supply (price and cost) as close to the patient as possible is the best way of controlling demand.

David Willetts, one of the intellectual architects of the 1990 reforms, pointed out that in the pre-reform system, choice was limited by bureaucracy and lack of information. But, he believed, it could be enhanced by the new contract-based system in which information would flow freely, allowing the choices made by individuals to be expressed through their GP. 'In future,' he wrote of the reforms, 'patients will be cherished because hospitals will want to win their custom.'[12]

The underlying philosophy of the reformers was based on a view of choice as a liberating force. It created efficiency, accountability and responsibility by elevating choice above direct participation in decision making. These dynamics have been characterized by Hirschman in a classic study as 'exit' and 'voice'. In systems such as the NHS, 'exit' refers to a quasi-commercial relationship, where a consumer can choose between different providers in a market. 'Voice' refers to a democratic model, where individuals have a say in how the system is run.[13] The reformed system elevated 'exit' over 'voice'.

According to John Spiers, a first wave trust chief executive: 'choice is a value with special transforming powers which can only be evolved within oneself.' He believes that it is precisely because the decisions in medicine are so complex and potentially so difficult – a traditional justification for the expert opinion of the medical profession – it can be left up to no one but the individual facing them to make them, wherever possible. A system that takes decisions out of the individual's hands is one that needs to be seriously questioned.[14]

On a broader scale, he believes that a system that reflects the power of choice, and which responds to it, is morally robust and economically fit. Thus, trust hospitals living on referral patterns, cherishing each customer as a source of income, are more wholesome than ones that do not analyse their activities and fail constantly to seek improvement.

Some doctors believe a choice-based system is already coming to pass. Adam Darkins is a neurosurgeon, turned director of public health of a community trust. He believes patients are dissatisfied with the information they receive from doctors about their conditions and the treatments they are offered. He contests arguments against giving patients more information about their conditions – that the data is too complex for them to understand and that they often prefer not to know full details. The changing nature of illness – from acute conditions that needed quick treatment and ruled out patient involvement to today's chronic illnesses, which give more time for reflection – have made involvement of the patient possible.

Darkins says there is evidence that patients who make decisions have more uniform rates of treatment.[15] He also believes that bringing patients into the relationship has benefits because it empowers them, but also that, due to the conservative views of patients, it is likely to decrease the costs of care. Others may argue the opposite: that if patients gain greater control in the decision making process, they will demand more and more treatment, and push costs up.

The patient may still be isolated without advice or help. The doctor must always be able to advise. It is a rebalancing that is called for, but it is vital that we keep a link between what we do and its consequences. The thousands of decisions taken by patients and doctors in partnership may not be anyone's business but those individuals' but their aggregate effect certainly is – particularly in the reformed health service – as it defines the public's use of the system.

However, the view that unbridled choice can have damaging consequences has gained influence since the early years of the 1990s. The concern is based on two propositions. The first is that choice undermines equity by giving some greater choice and power of exercising it than others. We shall examine this in a later section. The second is that it appears to undermine equity, and therefore is perceived to undermine a key justification for the system. This, in turn, gnaws at the feeling of serenity or well being at the base of the NHS and, ironically, has led to measures that inhibit choice.

Indeed, far from protecting and strengthening the precious institutions of British life, the market can damage them. One distinguished proponent of this view is the Oxford political philosopher John Gray. Gray's espousal of these ideas is interesting because for many years he held opposing views which influenced Thatcherite reformers. His ideas were important in the early 1980s, when he argued that British economic and social life had to be opened up to market forces if the country was to escape the impasse of trade unionism and corporatism that was the partner of economic stagnation.

Much of the defence of the application of free market economics continues to rely on the fear of a return to the 1970s. But Gray writes:

It is a general truth that, when they are disembodied from any context of common life, and emancipated from political constraints, market forces … work to unsettle communities and delegitimate traditional institutions. This is a truism, no doubt; but it expresses an insight – that, for most people, security against risk is more important than the enhancement of choice – that conservative parties and governments have forgotten. For many people, perhaps most, the largely illusory enhancement of choice through freeing up markets does not compensate for the substantial increase in insecurity it also generates.[16]

Gray's view expresses the importance of security – interpretable as Bevan's serenity – and suggests that the institutions which promote these feelings are extremely valuable. If markets do threaten the security – even the perception of the safety of the system that promotes that security – then they are doing harm to society and undermine the justification for the system as it stands.

The problem with choice and competition in health care is that they create, at least in the medium term, winners and losers in a system that exists to allow only winners. Thus choice may logically lead to the closure of hospitals that do not provide services of high quality and good value. In an extreme view of the effect of the market, one analyst predicted the number of trusts would decline after pressure from purchasers forced them out of the market place. Highly specialized services would become concentrated, providing expensive high-technology treatment to large populations – between 750 000 and a million people. The barriers between primary, acute and community services would break down to merge into new forms of service, federal chains of trusts would emerge, and the private sector would increasingly be allowed in to operate as a provider in the NHS. He wrote: 'The forces let loose, even by a managed market, will lead to a rapid concentration and restructuring of providers. Trusts will face the need for radical change. A large number will have to merge whilst others will simply close.'[17] In addition the radical new purchasers, fundholders, created a differential between patients, some of whom may be treated more quickly than others, and introduced the threat of cream skimming.

The very notion of purchasing suggests that there are differences to exploit. In a politicized service such as the NHS, where equity is its justification, such tendencies are easy to attack, if not caricature. In fact as we shall see, the choice-driven internal market has been forestalled at almost every level of the NHS, from the GP's surgery to Richmond House. But it is the perception that counts.

While Darkins and Spiers argue that the markets need to be given space to move, the arguments of Gray and others, have led to them being constrained in practice. Fear of market failure has become a self-fulfilling prophesy.

Problems with purchasing

Purchasing was to be the driving force of change, focusing on what patients needed rather than on what doctors wanted to provide. There are specific problems with the purchasing structure, however, which have required remedies that in turn have undermined the structure itself.

Fragmentation is a key dilemma. The purchaser/provider split, which defines interactions between buyers and sellers in the NHS and between purchasers and the private sector has, 'the potential to give rise to a further form of fragmentation, that is, the differential provision of services to different populations or groups of registrants.[18]

This is a paradox of the reforms. Their central thrust is to forge a link between doctors and budgets, to make the focus on the individual widen to the needs of the group, but their method of doing so is based only on individualist behaviour. The reforms have put faith in thousands of individual decisions, each with its own financial consequences, being aggregated and creating a more efficient and fair system than was there under the old planned one.

As the reforms unwound, there were examples of two-tierism recounted weekly in the papers: fundholding patients getting quicker service, IVF being available in some parts of the country but not others and so on. So, while we, as patients may never know whether the market would have worked or what it would have achieved, we are still left with a service that is at least perceived to be less equitable than before the reforms. We have the worst of both worlds.

Primary care

Many fundholders themselves believe that they have succeeded in their aims. In a recent study a comparison of the effectiveness of fundholding and non-fundholding schemes in achieving their goals was carried out. The study concluded: 'If one takes the success rate in those cases where the two groups had conceived of there being a problem we find a two thirds success rate for fundholders and a 40% success rate for non-fundholders.' In other words, the study concluded that fundholders were getting better results in dealing with their major concerns than non-fundholders – although fundholders were much better resourced.[19]

Critics are unconvinced. The primary worry is the effect on equity. They point to the tendency of fundholding to splinter local services, to undermine the sense of strategy and planning needed to commission services properly and to create two tierism. As one leading health analyst says: 'Put simply, there is no guarantee that the sum of multiple purchasing decisions will add up to the pattern of service provision appropriate to the needs of the population concerned.'[20]

There are similarities with the risk-pool problems faced by insurance systems. There has been considerable concern over the spread of this into fundholding – which has many of the characteristics of an insurance company, paying out on patients who 'claim' in the budget by presenting themselves with illnesses, and having to deal with the claims of a defined list of people for a defined list of treatments.

Bartlett and Le Grand state: 'There is an obvious danger of cream skimming by GP fundholders in their selection of patients for their lists.'[4] Newspaper stories like that covering a Newcastle practice, which asked people over 65, and therefore likely to be more costly, to register with another practice, confirm suspicions that such factors are at work – although hard evidence is not widespread.[21]

Consumer groups are also far from happy at what they see as 'mixing money and medicine'. A report by the Consumers Association found over two-thirds of GPs surveyed believed a two-tier service was in operation, giving doctors the incentive not to treat expensive patients or to refer for expensive conditions. It also expressed concern that fundholders were squeezing patients and patient groups out of the commissioning function and noted that fundholders were funded over-generously. In short, while saying fundholders themselves tended to like the scheme, it questioned the benefits fundholding was throwing up for patients. 'Choice may have increased in the NHS, but it seems to be choice for the GP, not for the consumers' it concluded.[22] As if to confirm the points, official figures show in July 1997 60% of health authorities had shorter waiting lists for fundholding patients – although 37% have shorter waits for non fundholders.[23]

Fundholding also corrupts the purchaser/provider split which lies at the heart of the internal market by making GPs providers. On the one hand the attempt to shift services away from hospitals is seen as positive; moving care into the community – on the other it may provide the fundholder with an incentive not to refer to a hospital when hospital treatment is necessary.

There is another question concerning fundholder intentions. Fundholders are permitted to keep the savings they make to invest in the 'benefit of their patients' and this controversially includes investment in their own practices. As one report stated, 60% of savings from schemes are used to invest in practice improvements, but 'it is not clear in what way this is a priority for the NHS, nor whether it is appropriate to invest public monies into private real estate.'[24]

Management of these shortcomings has gradually moved fundholding away from what was originally intended, towards the other models including 'commissioning' groups, where GPs influence the decision-making processes rather than through individual use of budgets. The movement has been spearheaded by GPs who are concerned by the equity implications of fundholding, in the belief that wider commissioning groups can maintain equitable distribution of resources while retaining purchasing muscle. As we shall see, commissioning groups and multi-funds have spread and often involve fundholders.[25] It is a development of the internal market that has been seized on by politicians, keen to make the new system acceptable.

Limits to the primary care market

Choice was intended to be a safeguard for the patient as well as the purchaser. At the entry point of the service, it was to allow patients to protect their interests by changing between GPs.

We have seen how the philosophical tide has turned against choice as an engine of change. This has followed through into everyday life in the NHS. Patients can theoretically change GPs but it is unclear how often this happens, or even if patients consider this to be an effective way of exercising choice. One survey reported: 'Most people change GP only when they move house, registering with the one closest to their home rather than shopping around.'[26] Once in the GP surgery the scope for choice diminishes as decisions are increasingly taken on a professional basis. So the re-orientation of the service to consumers may be illusory.

Consumer groups are sceptical of the difference the ability to choose a GP makes. Once within the surgery, mechanisms for GP choice are questionable. The extra-contractual referral system – which allows GPs to refer patients to providers that offer better service and quality outside their areas – has been attacked by managers, the medical profession and the Labour party as bureaucratic, costly and confusing.

In the absence of perfect choice, there are structural inflexibilities that are intended to protect both the fundholder and the patient from market forces. Only large practices could join – to dilute risk. The range of treatments that standard fundholders can purchase with their budgets – which average about £1.7 million per practice – was limited, so that only about 30% of hospital and community health care services were purchased by the fundholder – and this specifically excludes accident and emergency costs and treatments over £6000. Thus the risk they face is limited.

This can encourage moral hazard on the part of the fundholder – if a patient presents with a serious condition, there is an incentive to drive treatments up beyond £6000 to pass costs on to health authorities. There are other 'perverse incentives' – for example there is an incentive not to save too much of the budget in order to retain a reasonably high allocation in the following year.

In 1996 the number of patients per fundholder was reduced to 5000 for the standard model of fundholding. At the same time variations on the theme were encouraged by the government. Those with big practices and the will to press the advantages they perceived from the initial scheme were allowed to develop total purchasing pilots, where the GP took on a much larger budget to purchase all services – including accident and emergency and expensive cases like beta interferon in return for greater risk. There are currently more than 50 total purchasing pilots.[27]

Interestingly, total purchasing is not recognized in law. Pilot groups must themselves become subcommittees of their health authorities. They keep their original fundholding budgets individually, but pool the additional funds used to cover extra services such as accident and emergency, which come under control of the total purchasing group. These will be closely monitored by the health authority 'to ensure financial control and probity'. The line between the vulnerable but dynamic fundholder and the health authority – able to absorb large shocks – is blurred.[28]

Fundholding has not caused great shocks to the system for various reasons: the unwillingness of authorities to allow hospital trusts to go out of business, the fact that the shifts in purchasing patterns on trusts have not had as great an effect as was expected, and the willingness of fundholders to work with health authorities and experiment in many cases. And in overcoming the effects of shifts the nature of purchasing has changed. In fact the nature of purchasing has been changing constantly, moving away from a rigorous exchange towards a planning, commissioning role. Nevertheless, suspicion of fundholding has not subsided and the market continues to offer the worst of both worlds.

Legitimizing primary care

Despite the shortcomings of fundholding, the Conservative Government was committed to forging a new system through primary care to re-engineer the service away from costly producer dominance – a policy continued under Labour. Primary care cost less than hospitals and produced good results. Its strategy for a primary care-led NHS became more consensual as time wore on. By 1996 it was consulting primary care workers on how they saw the way forward – a tactic diametrically opposite to the introduction of fundholding in 1990.[29]

GPs had been active in modifying fundholding, mitigating the market, to their own purposes and the results were published in two White Papers last year, which stressed that the way forward was to be voluntary. They suggested a wide range of innovations in primary and secondary care, including the possibility of salaried GPs offering a greater range of services through practice contracts, and loosened the rigidity of the budgeting structure. A greater role for nurses was encouraged, getting more information to patients was supported and the need for measures to improve management was suggested. Piloting was to be encouraged.[30]

General practitioners themselves have been making their own responses to fundholding. In a survey by economists at the LSE, a difference in values between out-and-out fundholders and those experimenting with different forms such as commissioning and multifunds was expressed.

The team found that there was a wide variety of commissioning models. Some had control over budgets, defined responsibilities and wide use of information in decision making. At the other end of the spectrum some schemes had no control over budgets and little say in how decision making on commissioning care was carried through into practice.

The survey also found that different groups had wanted to achieve different things by joining the various schemes. Fundholders were concerned with small-scale, specific issues that affected them as practices; commissioning groups were concerned with wider scale ones. Fundholders had efficiency primarily in mind; commissioning groups were concerned about what fundholding did to equity and were working for greater influence while maintaining it.

The survey found that general practice was becoming greatly more influential, that fundholders and commissioning groups often worked together, and that they were both interested in redefining the boundaries of commission care. Crucially, it found that the two groups do different things well.[19]

Another recent report said: 'Fundholding has its place, but suddenly ... the number of models for gaining local ownership of purchasing decisions is growing almost daily.'[31] In a longer report, the same author outlined some of the diverse experiments in commissioning health care taking place, pointing to GPs' misgivings about fundholding, and found:

> Often based around GPs who preferred not to be fundholders, these models sought alternative ways of influencing the provision of services by trusts, ensuring that health services were sensitive to the needs of local people and were delivered on the basis of equity to all patients.

The report focused on six projects: in Belfast, Bromley, Dorset, Nottingham, Tynedale, Northumberland, and Wiltshire. In some cases, like Nottingham, the doctors involved were all non-fundholding. The Nottingham project involved some 200 GPs representing 68% of the city's population with an executive group that covered geographical boundaries roughly the same as social service authority areas. This group advised the

Nottingham Health Authority purchasing teams, thus linking it to the health authority and its broad commissioning strategy. The advice it gave was generally acted upon, and relations are described as excellent. The groups work alongside fundholding GPs and communicate via the local medical advisory committee.

Another example was in Bromley, where a clinical commissioning board was set up including nine elected GPs acting as clinical commissioning directors from their areas – ranging from 12 GPs covering 25 000 people, to 27 GPs with 61 000 patients – alongside the executive members of the health authority. The idea was to include all GPs, not only fundholders, in the commissioning process. The objectives of the board were described as achieving a balance between locality views and Bromley's health needs as a whole, information sharing, to build up relationships of trust between the health authority and GPs – not always historically sound. The report commented: 'Generally, the GPs feel that the health authority is listening and acting upon decisions made at meetings.'

The study summed up developments, saying: 'What is clear is that there is no single solution to the challenge of creating a primary care led NHS.' Key among the developments, was the relationship between the GP and the health authority. GPs were learning as well as working alongside the health authority, but the changes would not happen overnight – evolution, not revolution, was the keyword. Another factor was the team work between GPs and the sense of mutuality between health authorities and GPs – formerly the cause of much friction and power struggle.[31]

There is evidence that commissioning groups can overcome problems of fragmentation. According to Glennerster: 'Where a local monopoly provider exerts a powerful sway, more powerful collective action groupings may be optimal'.[19] Yet there are barriers to change, like the GP contract that gives a loose definition of what general medical services a GP must deliver. If this definition were tightened, argue some, so that a core package of services were defined for the GP, other workers could enter the primary care arena, making the services and the market more flexible and diverse.[32]

Despite the successes claimed by schemes like Nottingham, Bromley and Belfast, fundholders still claim the idea of commissioning GPs is just creating a 'talking shop'.

The only thing that really talks, is money, they say. Epsom-based Dr Tim Richardson, for example, says: 'The only way I can get change in my local hospital services is by threatening to withdraw funds. They aren't going to sit down and talk to me and listen.'[33]

However, it is by no means certain either that these alternatives are cheaper or more effective than in hospital. Primary care analyst Angela Coulter writes: 'It may be that primary care is not an acceptable substitute for secondary care in the popular imagination.' She adds: 'It is clear ... that achieving a shift in the balance of care is not going to be easy, and it is not even certain that it will prove cost effective. Changes are occurring, but their overall balance is at best marginal.' Coulter points out that there are limitations to the primary care led ethos – that the cost effectiveness of carrying out surgery in a primary care setting is questionable, that fundholders are not all up to the task of purchasing and that referral rates are still very variable across the country. The key, she believes, is in providing better facilities outside hospitals; facilities that do not, as yet, exist. Also: 'The shift will have to be actively managed if it is to proceed smoothly.'[34] And as that shift is encouraged by politicians it underlines the move away from pure market forces which has now established itself as political common ground.

Health authorities

Of the two types of purchaser the dominant and larger were health authorities. From the outset it was they who were given strategic responsibility for ensuring the health needs of their populations were met. They received cash-limited allocations from their regional health authorities (now offices of the NHS Executive) based on the size and profile of their populations to buy services.[35] In 1996 the original plan was altered with the merger with FHSAs to provide a more complete strategy for both primary and secondary care, and to bring forward the process of involving GPs in commissioning care.[36]

The purchasing system has been undermined by lack of progress over contracting. Contracts were the weapons by which purchasers would force efficiency out of providers in annual contracting rounds. Purchasers would look for their own efficiencies in service provision, above and beyond the 3% demanded annually by the Government's efficiency index.

The contracting system would also break one of the weaknesses of the old system, the so-called efficiency trap. Under the old health system, where health authorities ran hospitals, there was no incentive to treat greater numbers of patients. Since year-long budgets were set and allocated to health authorities, and passed on to their directly managed units, each extra patient was an added drain on these resources. So a hospital that was efficient and managed to treat more patients than another could end up being penalized. Contracts linking payment to volumes of patients treated or even to individual cases were envisaged by reformers, allowing money to follow patients, so making sure that greater volumes would not be penalized.

The system was let down by the form of the contracts. There are three types. In block contracts purchasers pay a sum of money per year for a defined range of services.

These were crude agreements that were insensitive to workload and type of treatment, making the tailoring of services to patient requirements almost impossible and loading risk on the side of the hospital. Cost and volume contracts involved purchasers paying an agreed price for a volume of work, with payments or deductions as appropriate. Cost per case contracts tied payment to the delivery of individual services to individual patients.

The market has struggled to operate properly because, although fundholders have been keen to use cost and volume contracts, the bulk of services purchased by health authorities has been through block arrangements. There has been some move towards 'sophisticated block' contracts – in which purchasers negotiated extra services with providers at marginal prices. These indicate there is some link between cost and volume, but it is limited.[37] A National Audit Office report in 1995 pointed to grave difficulties with the system of block contracts.[38] In addition the number of disputes has increased throughout the process.[39]

In the case of the block contract there is only a very crude link between demand and supply and what is actually delivered on a contract. The block contract does not link funds to patients going through the system. The efficiency trap is maintained.

There is also the question of 'moral hazard'. If there is a block contract there is no incentive for purchasers to keep down the number of referrals because they do not have to pay for them. On the other side of the divide, where hospital budgets are tight on block contracts, managers will seek to take cost per case patients – as we see in Chapter 4 where fundholding patients were preferred to non-fundholding ones.

Professor Ray Robinson, who contributed to a recent University of Birmingham study says:

There has certainly been an evolution in contracting in the NHS market. Sophisticated block contracts provide a floor and ceiling to the block, around which services are negotiated at marginal cost. There has been more stability between purchasers and providers than was originally planned. District health authorities contract with providers in much the same way as they did before the reforms. The relationships are still close. On the other hand there are some examples where at the margins of the contracting system there has been change in the nature of particular services. This is especially true of services like orthopaedics. Some health authorities are involved in this, but it is more likely to be fundholders.[40]

A report by the National Association of Health Authorities and Trusts stated the 1996–97 contracting round was 'generally regarded as the most difficult since the reforms'. The report pointed to an NHS being 'squeezed between increasing demand for services and modest financial growth', and said that the main concerns deriving from this were funding increased volumes of care. Funding pay increases was also a major problem. Finding all this within an annual 1.1% growth in the NHS budget to £42.49 billion while making the 3% efficiency saving was challenging, it said.[39]

Purchasers are aware of this, and as a result the course of the reforms is altering from the outright competitive model envisaged at the outset to a more planned model now.

As one analyst, who has surveyed purchasing plans throughout the UK, says:

> Most (though not all) commissioners put more emphasis on planning service provision than promoting competition: shaping the market rather than responding to it. Many health authorities recognise the danger that competition may lead to replication of services and is therefore not an efficient use of resources.'[41]

Provider strength

Another problem with the market is the structure of the pattern of hospitals inherited from Powell's hospital plan, and the resilience of hospitals themselves. One analyst says: 'A study of changing concentration ratios, that is the percentage of health authority spending focused on three or less providers, would show this to be rising steadily. In other words purchasers are being tied more tightly to a smaller number of acute providers.[42]

This reflects the undynamic nature of the purchaser/provider relationship, but also the power of the localized district general hospital (DGH) system to defend itself from the threat of service reconfiguration. In another paper, the same analyst states: 'Hospitals are the icons of health care, irrespective of their true powers they are perceived at least by politicians, and perhaps by the public, as close to sacred.'[43] Inefficient trusts have simply not been going out of business.

Attitudes to hospitals reinforce the feeling that purchasing has never really worked. The purchasing function did not gain sharp enough teeth to make enough of a difference. 'The management talent stayed in the hospitals' is a commonly repeated statement. And the geographical distribution of hospitals creates local monopolies that work against the market – particularly in the absence of small alternatives to the DGH.

In a study of the West Country Bartlett concluded: 'It is likely that the quasi-market will fail to operate in a competitive fashion in many local areas' – thanks to the small number of purchaser and providers – although in areas like London the greater amount of players will increase competition.[44]

John Redwood, former Secretary of State for Wales, found Wales to be an example of how geography could undermine the working of the market. Hospitals in Wales could cover vast areas without competition and therefore exist as monopolies:

> I found that when I arrived in Wales, the centralising culture had taken deep root. Many of the managers wanted to close Merthyr Hospital, they said it was too old. They had built the new Prince Charles Hospital in an adjacent valley. But it was well defended by the local people, who wanted to keep it open.

> The forces to close were very very strong, but I resisted them, and introduced a policy of no more closures of hospitals in Wales unless the community supported them. The argument was about choice. You can have a certain amount of choice within a district general hospital, but I think choice is maintained much better if you have a choice of institutions within a geographical area. The cottage hospitals provide that, and that is why I fought for them.[45]

Hospitals also have to maximize revenue. There is a built-in incentive for hospitals to view health care as the treatment of sickness, and downplay the role of public health. This reinforces the expensive medical model of health – one of the things the reforms specifically aimed to weaken.

Relationships with other hospitals, with the health authorities that contract with the trust to give it its income, with the GP fundholders who make up the rest of the purchasing ranks, who demand shorter waiting times for their lists, are set against this background.

For a start, purchasers will want to move their spending patterns away from the hospital sector – which currently absorbs such a high proportion of their budgets. They want to see waiting lists cut, they want the lowest prices, so if a hospital does have excess capacity purchasers want it used at marginal cost.

Several methods have been tried to break the deadlock caused by the insensitive contracting system. They are based around cracking open the service agreements between purchasers and providers, creating incentives to operate within given financial incentives and achieve quality and targets as well as enabling purchasers to track individual patients.

Box 3.2: Integrated care

Managing the costs of care by manipulating incentives has been tried in the USA, where Health Maintenance Organizations (HMOs) have proliferated. As their name suggests, HMOs start by persuading people to remain healthy and so keep down medical costs. Beyond that are a number of cost management techniques. HMOs state clearly what services their members are entitled to which usually involves restricting the choice of doctors, selecting hospitals to provide secondary care, emphasizing the importance of primary care and being rigorous about applying clinical guidelines to treatments they are willing to pay for. Dr Harry Burns, Director of Public Health at Greater Glasgow Health Board, believes the system could be adapted in this country.

In the USA they were used to controlling spiralling costs which were induced by the third party payment system. Doctors were paid on a fee-for-service basis giving them an incentive to inflate their incomes by providing more, often unnecessary, care. In the UK their use would be similar in terms of cost containment but the fee-for-service problem has never been the dominant reason.

HMOs have grown in number from about 400 in 1985 with 19 million subscribers to 1500 today, covering 50–55% of the US population. However, the evidence on whether they keep costs down is mixed as hospitals are adept at manipulating codes by which treatments are classified in order to receive payment for more expensive treatments than those that were in fact required or performed. There are equity problems too because the organization's focus is clearly on efficiency and cost saving regardless of the relative range and access to service on offer to its patients.[3]

In Britain there is already one cost containment mechanism in place – the GP. But many purchasers believe the split between primary and secondary care, coupled with the clumsy contracting system, is undermining its ability to deliver the efficiency it could. If care was integrated there would be an overall interest in keeping costs down, and the conflict between cost containing GP fundholders and hospitals would be replaced by a more strategic view.

The virtues of integrated or managed care are also being explored in Manchester, where similar public health problems pose similar pressures on the city's health budget. Neil Goodwin, Chief Executive of Manchester Health Authority says: 'At the moment we contract to deliver a broad spectrum of care to the population. It is not an easy system to manage. The expectation is that in future we will look to place a contract for a particular service with a particular provider, who will then subcontract throughout the system. So if we contracted with a hospital to provide diabetes care, they will be responsible for contracting with GPs and community services to deliver the whole package of care to patients in Manchester. At the moment the separate components do not come together at all. And it is not a patient focused system – it is currently only GP fundholders who purchase for the individual.'

Goodwin continues: 'In managed care systems, purchasers will expect to have control over the types of treatment they pay for so they will have a hand in drawing up treatment protocols. Providers who move out of line will have to be controlled. Whatever systems we use, they should be centred on the patient and we should be able to track the patient through the system, allowing us to assess the quality of care we are giving and see what effects the system has on costs. The Manchester system is being pioneered for several services – diabetes, coronary heart disease, depressive illness, management of stroke, children's health.'

Roger Johnson is a GP who also works for Manchester Health Authority on the managed care projects. 'Take diabetes,' he says, 'When caring for diabetics there is almost always a partnership between primary and secondary care. But the problem is that there is very compartmentalized management at the moment. There are the GPs – in Manchester there are around 100 practices, with something around 300 GPs. Then there are community nurses managing and visiting diabetics. They belong to Manchester Community Healthcare Trust. Then there are specialist medical services for diabetics who need to come in and see a diabetologist, who is based at the district hospital closest to the patient. There are three in Manchester. Then there are the more specialist services which may be needed, provided by a more limited number of tertiary sites. There are also the community ophthalmologists for the many who develop sight problems. This is a very complicated system. It creates a management black hole where everything is somebody else's responsibility and nobody can be held to account for anything. Part of the problem is the contracting system. We do block contracts and cost and volume. So we can't gauge what we spend on diabetes each year.'

As part of the managed care initiative, Dr Johnson is piloting an accreditation scheme in Manchester to help with the quality of the diabetics services on offer. He days: 'The patient is the stick. Patients should be told what to expect from diabetes services, based on the standards drawn up under the scheme. They will also be told about the educational services they can expect and what the overall pattern of care should look like for the next few years. They will be told what complications we would be trying to prevent and how we would go about doing that. If they are not being given the care that is described they can also ask to change the

> primary or the secondary care provider. They take their funds with them, so the money really does follow the patient and the service becomes patient-orientated.
>
> Interviews with Neil Goodwin, August 1996, Roger Johnson, August 1996 and Harry Burns, August, 1996.

These are known variously as integrated care or managed care systems and are modelled on examples such as health maintenance organizations (HMOs) in the USA, which use a detailed set of specific agreements between insurance companies and providers to ensure quality and financial control are exerted throughout. Examples in the UK are growing. Both Manchester and Glasgow are experimenting, as is a GP surgery in Lyme Regis for example, which self-consciously calls itself an HMO.[46]

The systems for managing care and costs in Britain are underdeveloped. Structurally, the NHS has a great advantage over American systems in the gatekeeping GP who, as we have seen, keeps costs down. Nevertheless, Robert Royce, a manager who has worked in both systems, points out that neither fundholders nor health authorities have the sophisticated management techniques in place that could lever in efficiencies after referral by GPs.[47]

Royce runs through a series of payment management systems that American health maintenance organizations have used to limit the formerly open-ended exposure of US insurers to health care costs. These include fee caps, capitation of primary care, different hospital payment management systems including specific payments systems for specific treatments – known as 'diagnostic related groups'. These techniques will be more familiar to private managers than NHS ones in the UK because the private system has had to emulate the American lead in the absence of effective gatekeepers and the consequent pressures for moral hazard.

The NHS has lagged – almost complacently – behind. There is little wish to analyse the inputs and outputs of treatment. US managers often ask Royce: 'How are you hoping to operate a market successfully when you have no clarity on your currency?' The NHS has no management over how the services a purchaser pays for are used.

Analysis of risk pools is also underdeveloped in the NHS, with little integration between fragmented purchasing agencies. Coupled with the refusal to become involved in patient tracking – despite attempts to instil this in the system through fundholding – the lack of risk pool co-ordination leads to wide variations in referral rates, treatment and costs around the country. Royce argues that fundholding should be geared around capitation funding which would underpin clear and logical reimbursement systems.

But Royce points out that although fundholders have grown in number, they are generally squeezed out of the contracting process, which remains driven by health authorities and trusts, looking to guarantee the lions share of their contracts each year before moving on to fundholders at the margins. It is this fact that allows the system to retain its instinctive conservatism and fear of change.[47]

Private sector in the market

The relationship between the State and the private sector is *ad hoc* and fluid. It is influenced by the regulatory regime – whether and on what terms private insurers may operate – and by the working conditions and pay structures of the medical profession, which are determined by the State and which have effects on private sector costs. In addition, the attitude of the Government to taxing both subscribers to health insurance and the companies themselves have impacts on demand and supply respectively.

The current private sector relationship with the NHS has been characterized by two main factors: time and amenity – higher standards of 'hotel' services, private rooms, televisions and so on.

There has been considerable growth since the 1980s on the 'provider' side – private hospitals supplied 19.8% of all UK hospital-based treatment in 1995, compared with 9.9% nine years earlier. At the beginning of last year there were 224 independent hospitals with operating theatres in the UK, with a total of 11 210 beds. There are some 15 groups that operate hospitals on a significant scale, led by BUPA, which has 29 hospitals with 1704 beds, and General Healthcare Group which has 25 with 1543, down to single hospital minnows.[48]

The growth has slowed since. This is accounted for by the slowdown in growth of private medical insurance and a slowdown in another area of private sector activity – the nursing home – due to community care reforms. The total value in 1995 of private supply was £5.4 billion, broken down into £1.9 billion in acute services and £3.4 billion for nursing home care. The bulk of acute care income is earned through medical, surgical and outpatient work – £1.2 billion in 1995. These figures compare with a total NHS hospital budget of £21.4 billion for 1993–94, of which acute care makes up £10.3 billion. These figures have been projected forward to give an estimated total hospital budget of £21.7 billion, of which acute care takes up £13.1 billion for 1996–97.[49]

One study cautions that the private sector is vulnerable to continued contraction if the NHS maintains the improvements in performance, and the public see waiting times falling in future.[5]

In general, contracts between NHS purchasers and the private sector have been limited to ancillary services like pathology and imaging services, and for long-term care in nursing homes although in high demand specialties like orthopaedics there is cross-over too. Laing estimates that the total amount of GP fundholder business within the private sector accounts for about 2% of the £1.3 billion annual turnover.[48]

In addition to this, the NHS is itself gaining a larger slice of the market to treat patients who have private medical insurance. The NHS has taken back some 4% of private patient market share in 1995 compared with the low point of its activity in 1988. In 1994–95, NHS revenue from private patients totalled £209 million. In 1995–96 the figure was expected to be £230 million.[44]

While the fluctuations in future demand for private medical insurance may depend on perceptions of the overall performance of the NHS in the public mind, the provision of paybeds actively to treat private patients is an area where market share is highly competitive. In 1996, for example, BUPA launched a new health fund, which sought to encourage longer term relationships with its subscribers, allowing credits to be carried over from one year to the next to the value of 8% of the insurance premium. This is intended to lock subscribers into the BUPA scheme and to increase loyalty. As part of the deal, however, the subscribers are encouraged to use one of a list of 150 hospitals on the scheme's list, which provide discounts to BUPA that would in turn fund the credit scheme to policy-holders. BUPA used the scheme to act against the trend towards NHS treatment of private patients by excluding NHS hospitals from the list. Newspaper coverage of the decision was interesting – painting the decision by BUPA as a threat to the NHS. Some papers called the move a £200 million cash threat to NHS revenues. Similar arrangements are prolif-erating across private health care organizations and, as Laing comments, 'network' schemes are the most significant new development as private health care companies try to maintain margins by securing low cost treat-ment.[50]

The BUPA move was an attempt to deal with what had become an express threat from the NHS as independent hospitals looked to maximize their revenues. So, far from creating more business in the form of referrals from purchasers, the reforms seemed to be taking business away from the private sector with providers taking advantage of a lucrative market using their facilities to beat private hospitals.

Of the 3000 pay beds in the NHS, the most significant are those within dedicated pay bed units in hospitals, numbering some 1400.

Dedicated units have private rooms, better catering, televisions and so on. In other words, not only are they offering the primary advantage over the NHS – queue jumping – they are also providing the higher-standard facilities that are associated with the private sector. According to Laing & Buisson they rose from 74 units with 1376 beds in 1995 to 77 units with 1385 beds in 1996.

With the rise in the number of units came a rise in the amount of revenue brought into the NHS by this avenue. According to the Monopolies and Mergers Commission this doubled to £150 million between 1989 and 1992.[48,51]

Norwich Union – a private insurer with no hospitals – believes pay beds provide an important counter to the power of private hospitals. One senior manager believes without them private insurers would be in a worse monopoly situation than public purchasers:

> Private hospitals have been very good at setting themselves some distance away from each other – giving themselves a series of geographical monopolies. Patients would rather go to their local hospital than anywhere else, so if a private insurer did not have pay beds, he would have to choose the local private hospital. The only way at getting at what is a clear local monopoly situation is to have pay bed units.[52]

His views are echoed in a report by the Monopolies and Mergers Commission into private medical services. It states:

> The market for private medical services is highly imperfect. Most patients want to be treated in a local hospital. For this reason the private medical services market may be considered (with the exception of London and a few other dense urban areas) as a series of local markets in which the choice of consultant or hospital may be limited.[51]

Thus, in a mirror image of the way private sector hospitals were expected to help break the monopoly of NHS trusts after the introduction of the purchaser/provider split, public sector hospitals are there to help break the monopoly of private ones. The major difference is that in the latter case, it is clearly working. Norwich Union developed policies directing patients into NHS trust pay bed units in order to encourage trusts to develop their units, and to realize that there was a good market for private patients coming from the private insurers that were not also providers. The figures quoted above show it is working, and BUPA's response shows, probably, that it is hurting.

There have been accusations that pay beds are not in fact profitable, and that trusts are cross-subsidizing them in an attempt to win market share from the private sector. These concerns were addressed in a report by National Economic Research Associates (NERA) commissioned by

Norwich Union, which concluded that in four out of the five cases studied, pay beds were indeed profitable. This proved the point Norwich Union wanted to make – that pay beds were a legitimate part of the market and should be available for operators like themselves in order to move away from the concentrated market of providers like BUPA and BMI.[53]

The *ad hoc* relationship between public and private sectors could be formalized to make everyone aware of who does what. This has implications for the fundamental questions in health policy: the balance between efficiency and equity, the accountability of the system, and how services should be rationed.

A managed market

The market was introduced to bring in efficiency, but the market itself had to be managed. At the top level, the problems posed by political interference in the new system dated back to the mid 1980s, when Victor Paige resigned as chairman of the new, supposedly powerful NHS management board. Later, he wrote that ministers took all the important decisions because the NHS was surrounded by such high political pressure.[54]

The market was in effect shackled by the 'steady state' exerted on it by ministers in the first two years of reform. Contracts were to be analysed carefully and damaging effects limited, particularly in the run-up to the 1992 election. Chris Ham writes:

> The aim was to manage the market in the initial stages in order to avoid harmful instability. But as the reforms progressed the Government grip relaxed only slightly. Decisions on reconfiguring hospital services particularly in London were postponed and fudged by a leadership transfixed by adverse publicity. A series of definitions of how a market in theory differed from its application to the NHS followed from a succession of health secretaries, first William Waldegrave, who emphasized the ability to compare performance engendered by a market, and second by Virginia Bottomley who extended the argument, pointing to the information that had been made available by reform.[55]

Making the market politically acceptable sends confusing signals to those who are operating within it, obstructs the logical methods of reforms, reinforces the power groups and blurs the sense of mission that managers, particularly purchasers, need in order to alter the system and to make it, in their view, affordable.

There were other pressures. At the local level, the national waiting list initiative, introduced by Virginia Bottomley in 1993 is among the most recent. It forced purchasers and providers alike to focus on one element of their service, constraining their ability to model services around other local determinants of need.

One senior manager at a teaching hospital says:

> This was a particular obsession of the department. I have never seen anything set so much as a high priority as the requirement to get waiting lists down to 12 months in the NHS. For example there is a great conflict in the desire to reduce waiting lists from the 18 months and the provision of a fully functioning and efficient accident and emergency system. The two are of the highest priority, but this insistence on the waiting lists diverted funds – more doctors and beds have to be used.[56]

Chris Ham has emphasized, through the statements of succeeding ministers Waldegrave, Bottomley and Dorrell that competition is dead, if not dying. They began to stress a shift towards longer term co-operation and planning. At local level, while fundholders were busy making competition work, its utilization among health authorities was patchy.

A new agenda began to emerge. 'Contestability' has been used as a way of explaining the system, subtly altering the word from its original meaning – a market that works because it is contestable – to being a hybrid between planning and competition which maintains the threat of moving contracts elsewhere, while looking to build co-operative relationships. 'In a contestable health service it is the possibility that contracts may move that creates an incentive within the system, rather than the actual movement of contracts.[55] But is this all possible? Does it make sense? If threats are not carried out, people cease to believe in them and the cosiness of a planned system returns. So will contracts have to be removed, rather like nineteenth century admirals sacrificed – 'pour decourager les âutres'? The question is, does the fact that only one trust has gone out of business mean that the market is not working. Has this new contestability undermined it?

Box 3.3: The hospital manager

The hospital managers' view of reform comes from a key player in them, Peter Griffiths. Now head of the management college at the King's Fund, he was deputy to Sir Duncan Nichol throughout the period in which the plans for reform were drawn up, and the hospital led the way as one of the 57 first-wave trusts. 'After six years, if I was marking them out of 10, I would have given them 6', he says.

Griffiths continues: 'There are five areas I would judge them in – did they improve management, did they produce better information about costs and how health services are performing, do we have more transparency and openness about the decisions being made on priorities and efficiency, do we deliver better services to the individual, and do we have a more motivated work force?'

Under the first heading, Griffiths awards eight out of ten points. He says: 'Management is now much more focused on the right things. For example, providers know what they must focus on – efficiency – and health authorities focus on populations. And there is broadly speaking a better system for allowing judgements to be made about performance.'

He also says the information available to decision makers in health care – either managers or clinicians – has improved since 1989, but there is still a long way to go. he awards six out of ten under this heading.

He says the reforms have encouraged a much more open debate about certain issues. 'Take rationing,' he says:

The fact that health authorities are publishing priorities for their populations shows that these issues are being talked about. Within hospitals there are other issues. There is the view that health managers should not get involved with making rationing decisions, that these should be left to doctors. I believe this is not the right point of view, and that more information is needed to create a framework for decisions. We need to build on what is happening already. I would say six out of ten.

As for what the citizen has got out of it all, I would mark that slightly lower, at five. People have had to wait shorter times since the reforms came in and that is good. But others would say that could happen irrespective of reforms – you just need to put more money in to hire the doctors to do it. There is also evidence that the free flow of patients has not really worked out, and that, because of the contract system – and the use of block contracts – that people in fact have less choice than they had before.

As for morale within the service, I would say four out of ten. People within the service simply have not seen the benefits.

Interviews with Peter Griffiths, July/September 1996.

Box 3.4: The politician

Stephen Dorrell believes the time has come for closer co-operation within the context of the internal market that has been set up. He says that the purchaser/provider system has created greater information for politicians and managers to be able to run the system. But it has not dictated that the system should be run as a red-in-tooth-and-claw, competitive marketplace.

Trusts going out of business is not really the point. What happens is that providers offer to provide a certain quality of service at a certain volume to a purchaser. There may be two or three options in an area. One of them offers a better value solution than the others, and that one is chosen. This does not mean it is about a struggle for existence between hospitals. It is about delivering particular services in particular areas. There should be sufficient stability in the system to allow the purchaser to decide that if the service would be better delivered by two hospitals collaborating or merging their operations, that might be the way forward.

This ignores the fact that there is no better way of judging whether a service should be funded than if it is used.

Interview with Stephen Dorrell, November 1996.

Labour

The Government claims to have abolished the internal market. When he launched the White Paper that signalled its demise in December 1997, Frank Dobson said: 'Today we are sweeping away the internal market and replacing it with a system of integrated care that puts doctors and nurses in the driving seat.' But the White Paper itself stated: 'In paving the way for the new NHS the Government is committed to building on what has worked, but discarding what has failed.' It added: 'There are some sound foundations on which the new NHS can be built. Not everything about the old system was bad.'[57] In fact, Labour's White Paper of 1997 has more in common with the Conservative one of 1989 that launched the internal market reforms than Dobson would care to admit.

The starting points are the same. Both duck the fundamental funding issues – is 7.1% of GDP really an adequate amount to be spending on our health care? Both therefore advocate supply side reform over tougher measures like charging, splitting out health taxes or expanding private care. Like Stephen Dorrell's White Paper in 1996, Frank Dobson dismisses the possibility that demographic, technological and expectational demands will push health costs to unsustainable levels. 'The Government rejects this analysis,' it states, continuing: 'the pressures on the NHS are exaggerated. Indeed they have always been exaggerated.' As I argue later, it would be wrong to concentrate entirely on funding issues ignoring supply side reform. But there needs to be a balance struck between the two which has proved too bold a political move for both Conservatives and Labour since Margaret Thatcher started her reforms with Roy Griffiths. Both 'solutions' therefore sell themselves on offering a better service to 'consumers', while levering in efficiencies to a grossly inefficient system. Thus 1989's title *Working for Patients* finds an echo in 1997's blandishment that it is 'tailoring the NHS to meet the needs of individual patients.'

With such similar starting points it should not be surprising that the solutions offered by both parties have striking likenesses. Indeed, as we have noted elsewhere, the protestations of Labour about the evils of the internal market may be so loud because they have no better vision of their own. The fact that they are maintaining the purchaser/provider split and the 'contestability' of the system really means they have made no fundamental ideological shift at all.

This is not to say the Government is not making changes. It is in fact developing the system it inherited in some interesting ways. Some are useful, some are harmful. There are several points here. The first is already made: the rhetoric of abolition hides the reality of development of the system it inherited. The second is that that system could not itself be called a market because the market mechanism – the purchaser/provider split – was encumbered by the structural and political obstacles noted in this chapter. Third, flowing from this, the specific measures outlined in the White Paper are not so much abolishing an iniquitous market mechanism as evolving the strategies for managing that mechanism which have emerged since it was created in 1991. On examination, those measures themselves could further undermine the limited efficiencies that the limited market itself was able to deliver up until now. Finally, there is the strong possibility that by 1999, ten years after Thatcher launched her market reforms, they will have proved not to have solved the pressing questions of demand for health care that they so cleverly avoided. The market will have bought politicians ten years and seen the NHS through to its 50th, but the questions that faced it within months of its creation will still be there. Do we spend enough on it?

These factors are most evident in the core proposal of the 'New NHS' – primary care groups. These are an evolution of the commissioning groups already discussed in this chapter and they will replace fundholding. The Government envisages groups of up to 50 GPs commissioning care using 'unified budgets' which combine money for both hospital and drug costs. There are four 'steps' in the evolution of these groups – at the lowest level they will work with health authorities to commission services, at their most advanced they will form primary care trusts with management of millions of pounds for the commissioning of care from hospitals and the provision of much of it themselves. They thus extend the corruption of the purchaser/provider split which was noted under fundholding. Health authorities will find their responsibilities wither as primary care evolves, finally existing only as monitors of performance and commissioners of highly specialized services.

The primary groups portray the key characteristics of the Labour strategy. They are intended to carry on the process of legitimising the primary care sector as the basis of the NHS commissioning system which was begun under the Conservative 'primary care-led NHS'. In the words of the paper they will 'mean fewer commissioners with more clout', reducing the total number from 3600 to as few as 500. They are also intended to rid the system of the fragmentation and two tierism that have been present since before the market, but which have been over stated by Labour in opposition since 1989.

The Government also claims that, along with other White Paper reforms, they will reduce bureaucracy as part of the White Paper's grand aim of stripping out £1 billion of paperchase costs within the lifetime of the 1997 Parliament. The groups will also have a cap on their management costs. But the arguments do not quite stack up. For a start, the new commissioning groups are themselves forming another layer of bureaucracy and they continue on a theme Labour used in opposition – anti-managerialism. The problem with this now they are in power is that although management costs may be high, they are vital for increasing efficiency. In addition, as the Audit Commission made clear in its fundholding analysis, doctors – and this can be extended to commissioners as well as fundholders – do not necessarily make good managers.

In addition, as Glennerster noted, fundholders and commissioners do different things well. Commissioning has positive effects on equity and fragmentation issues, but may limit the incentives created by fundholding. Moreover, it is not necessarily possible to force them to co-operate. As one commentator notes: 'The crux of the new reforms is this: can groups of GPs, organised in primary care groups, take on the innovative role of GP fundholders, or will they just become junior health authorities?'[58]

The Government's attitude to hospital trusts displays the same features as its policy on primary care. Theoretically, trusts are still subject to market contestability – although this is weakened by the need for three prior processes of investigation before a commissioner can switch contracts. The workings of the market will be further weakened by lengthening annual contracts to three or five year health improvement programmes. This may have positive effects in reducing costs but it undermines the incentives to save. Time will tell if that is an acceptable compromise.

The focus on gearing services around specific conditions or groups of patients announced in the White Paper is positive – pilots around the country have shown that such 'integrated care' systems are often very effective. But what is worrying is the lack of detail on how these agreements will work. The use of information and the sensitivity of agreements between purchasers and providers to the measurement of performance is crucial in maintaining the incentives for efficiency and quality that the Government emphasizes. As we have seen, crude measures such as block contracts can destroy attempts at analysis in any system. As the Economist notes: 'The Government says proposals such as these will mean more co-operation and less competition in the health service. But lumping doctor's budgets together and telling them to co-operate by no means guarantees co-operation. The Government also wants hospitals to compete less and co-operate more... But again it is making these vague noises about ending competition just as evidence is emerging that it actually works.'[59]

Finally, there are other problems. The Government has set up a number of national initiatives – a National Institute for Clinical Excellence and a Commission for Health Improvement are two examples. These could have wholly beneficial effects in levering up standards, the first by pressurizing doctors into using up-to-date and proven treatments, and the second by using a national performance framework and a range of comparative cost and quality indicators which replace the purchaser efficiency index. But as the *Financial Times* warned: 'The worry must be that the pendulum will swing too far the other way towards planning and control. The proposed Commission for Health Improvement – an NHS inspectorate armed with interventionist management powers – could all too easily become the dead hand of bureaucracy.'[60]

Labour continues to criticise the market, but the reality is that it has retained its key feature. At the same time it is falling into the same mistakes as made by the Conservatives. It recognizes the analytical value of the market, but is frightened of the consequences for equity and solidarity of letting it rip. It will therefore manage it, just as the Conservatives did – in Labour's case through commissioning GPs and by insisting on long-term contracts. These threaten to undermine further the purchaser/provider split's ability to provide greater flexibility and effectiveness to just the same extent as Conservative management has hitherto done.

The Government has exaggerated the danger of the internal market while advocating policies that are already taking shape. It is, in short, using the NHS to make political points. There is nothing new in this. But there should be an attempt to move on from the past Government's mistakes. Those mistakes, as we shall now see, have effected the whole shape of the system, from conceptual issues like lack of accountability and funding through to failure to address hospital reconfiguration, new treatment and training methods and rationing.

References

1 Labour Party (1995) *Renewing the NHS*. Labour Party, London; *Labour to cut NHS bureaucracy by scrapping Tories market*, speech by Alan Milburn on July 1 1996; Interview with Chris Smith, December 16 1996.
2 McGuire A, Fenn P and Mahew K (1991) Econometric analysis of national health expenditure, in A McIntyre (ed) *Providing Healthcare: the economics of alternative systems*. Oxford University Press, Oxford.
3 Appleby J (1992) *Financing Healthcare in the 1990s*. Open University Press, Buckingham.
4 Bartlett W and Le Grand J (1993) The theory of quasi markets, in J Le Grand and W Bartlett (eds) *Quasi Markets and Social Policy*. Macmillan, Basingstoke.
5 Clark G, Hockley T and Smedley I (1995) *The Insurance of Medical Risks*. Policy Analysis Centre, London.
6 BMA (1980) *The Handbook of Medical Ethics*. BMA Publishing Group, London.
7 Griffiths R (1983) *NHS Management Inquiry*. DHSS, London; Ranade W (1994) *A Future for the NHS?* Longman, Harlow.
8 Edwards B (1993) *The National Health Service: a manager's tale 1946–92*. Nuffield Provincial Hospitals Trust, London.
9 Edwards B (1993) *Op. Cit.*; Ham C (1992) *Health Policy in Britain*. (3rd ed.) Macmillan, Basingstoke, p. 35.
10 Enthoven A (1985) *Reflections on the Management of the National Health Service*. Nuffield Provincial Hospitals Trust, London.
11 Taylor D (1995) *Healthcare, Health Promotion and the Future General Practice*. Nuffield Provincial Hospitals Trust, London.
12 Willetts D (1989) *A Conservative NHS*. Conservative Political Centre, London, p. 44.
13 For a discussion of the alternatives of 'voice' and 'exit' see Hirschman A (1970) *Exit, Voice and Loyalty: responses to decline in firms, organizations and states*. Harvard University Press, Cambridge, MA.
14 Spiers J (1997) *Who Owns Our Bodies? making moral choices in health care*. Radcliffe Medical Press, Oxford.
15 Darkins A (1996) *Shared Decision Making in Health Care Systems*. Working paper. Unpublished.
16 Gray J (1994) *The Undoing of Conservatism*. Social Market Foundation, London. For an exposition of the value of choice and markets to institutions such as the health service see Willetts D (1994) *Civic Conservatism*. Social Market Foundation, London.
17 Newchurch Health Briefing (1993) *Strategic Change in the NHS 1 – unleashing the market*. Newchurch & Co, London.

18 Harrison S and Lachman P (1996) *Towards a High Trust NHS*. Institute of Public Policy Research, London.

19 Glennerster H, Cohen A and Bovell V (1996) *Alternatives to Fundholding*. London School of Economics and Political Science Welfare State Programme discussion paper WSP/123, London.

20 Ham C (1996) Population-centred and patient-focused purchasing. *Millbank Quarterly.* **74**: 2.

21 Fletcher D (1996) GPs asked pensioner patients to move on. *Daily Telegraph.* April 19.

22 Hoey A (1995) GP fundholding: mixing money and medicine. *Consumer Policy Review.* **5**: Sept/Oct.

23 Murray I (1997) Fundholder patients must join the queue. *Times.* July 17.

24 Stewart-Brown S, Gillam S and Jewell T (1996) The problems of fundholding. *BMJ.* **312**: 1311–12.

25 For history and background to GP commissioning see Singer R (ed.) (1997) *GP Commissioning: an inevitable evolution*. Radcliffe Medical Press, Oxford.

26 Consumers Association (1995) The good GP guide. *Which? Way to Health:* August.

27 NHS Executive (1994) *Towards a Primary Care Driven NHS: developing NHS purchasing and GP fundholding*. NHS Executive Briefing BNO No. 1, 19 October.

28 Smith R (1996) An introduction to total purchasing. The total purchasing group: relations between individual GPs, practices and the health authority; and Contracting for change, in R Smith, F Butler and M Powell (eds) *Total Purchasing: a model for locality commissioning*. Radcliffe Medical Press, Oxford, pp. 1–4, 14–23, 37–57.

29 Dorrell S (1996) *Primary care: the future*. NHS Executive, London.

30 Secretary of State for Health (1996) *The National Health Service: a service with ambitions* (Cmnd 3425). HMSO, London; Secretary of State for Health (1996) *Primary Care: delivering the future* (Cmnd 3512). HMSO, London.

31 Shapiro J, Smith J and Walsh N (1996) *Approaches to Commissioning: the dynamics of diversity*. NAHAT, Birmingham.

32 Ham C (1996) A primary health care market? *BMJ.* **313**: 127–8.

33 Interview with Dr Tim Richardson, June 1996.

34 Coulter A (1996) Shifting the balance between primary and secondary care, in M Peckham and R Smith (eds) *Scientific Basis of Health Services*. BMJ Publishing Group, London; Coulter A (1995) Shifting the balance from secondary to primary care. *BMJ.* **311**: 115–23.

35 Ranade W (1994) *Op Cit.*

36 NHS Executive (1995) Briefing note BN 35/95.

37 Raftery J, Robinson R, Mulligan J-A *et al.* (1996) Contracting in the NHS quasi market. *Health Economics.* **5**: 353–62.

38 National Audit Office (1995) *Contracting for Acute Health Care in England*. HMSO, London.

39 NAHAT (1996) *The 1996/97 Contracting Round*. NAHAT, Birmingham.

40 Interview with Professor Ray Robinson, July 1997.

41 Redmayne S (1996) *Small Steps, Big Goals: purchasing policies in the NHS*. Centre for the Analysis of Social Policy, NAHAT, Birmingham.
42 Newchurch Health Briefing (1994) *Strategic Change in the NHS 2. Investing for health – future of purchasing*. Newchurch & Co, London.
43 Newchurch Health Briefing (1994) *Strategic Change in the NHS 3. Acute Services – a prognosis for the millennium*. Newchurch & Co, London.
44 Bartlett W and Harrison L (1993) Quasi markets and the National Health Service reforms, in J Le Grand and W Bartlett (eds) *Quasi Markets and Social Policy*. Macmillan, Basingstoke.
45 Interview with John Redwood, November 1996.
46 Interviews with Neil Goodwin, Chief Executive, Manchester Health Authority, August 1996; Harry Burns, Director of Public Health, Greater Glasgow Health Board, August 1996; Dr Barry Robinson, GP, Lyme Regis, September 1996; *Manchester Health Authority Progress Report* (1996) on developing integrated care, unpublished.
47 Royce R (1997) *Managed care: practice and progress*. Radcliffe Medical Press, Oxford.
48 Laing W (1996) *Laing's Review of Private Healthcare, 1996/97*. Laing & Buisson, London.
49 Secretary of State for Health and Chief Secretary to the Treasury (1996) *The Government's Expenditure Plans 1996–97 to 1998–99* (Cmnd 3212). HMSO, London; Cocks R and Bentley R (1996) *Government Spending: the facts*. Databooks, Reading.
50 Interview with William Laing, July 1997.
51 Monopolies and Mergers Commission (1994) *Private Medical Services* (Cmnd 2452). HMSO, London.
52 Interview, July 1996.
53 National Economic Research Associates (1995) *Are Paybeds Profitable?* Norwich Union Healthcare, London; Fletcher D (1996) NHS to earn more from paybeds than BUPA. *Daily Telegraph*. March 25; Brindle D (1996) Private bed profit for NHS trusts. *Guardian*. March 25.
54 Ham C (1992) *Health Policy in Britain*. (3rd ed.) Macmillan, Basingstoke, p. 153.
55 Ham C (1997) *Management and Competition in the NHS*. (2nd ed.) Radcliffe Medical Press, Oxford.
56 Interview with Purchasing Manager, Guy's Hospital, September 1996.
57 Secretary of State for Health (1997) *The New NHS* (Cmnd 3807). HMSO, London.
58 Buckby S (1997) Some Conservative reforms will remain intact. *Financial Times*. December 10.
59 The Economist (1997) *Killing the cure*. November 8, p. 34.
60 Leader (1997) *Financial Times*. December 10.

4 Doctor knows best

Why is going to the doctor so different from going to a lawyer to seek legal advice, a building society or garage? The decisions we take in those places are complex – should we sue, what kind of mortgage are we to have, will we need a new clutch? We may know little or nothing about the products on offer but we expect to have some say in the decision making and some come back if the quality of what we pay for is not up to scratch. We expect some accountability of lawyer, lender or mechanic.

There are arguments about methods of teaching. However, our understanding of what we expect from education and from schooling is good enough for us to be confident about measuring how well it is being done. In this respect education leads health by a wide margin. Whereas, in the past, league tables for schools based on exam results have, like hospital tables, stopped short of asking the crunch question – 'who are the bad teachers?' – there is now a new drive towards establishing real accountability, to identify poor individuals and to root out bad practice.

There are no plans for the same power of sanction over doctors. We do not feel able to hold doctors to account. Why? Is it because we are more frightened to take decisions affecting our health than we are over our livelihoods?

Part of the answer is to do with the mystery surrounding medicine, and the medicalization of health care. The doctor interprets our unwellness as disease, categorizing it as something he or she understands. As one GP says: 'Illness is what the patient has on the way to see the doctor and a disease is what they have on the way home.'[1] We have gone from being unwell and uncertain to being diseased but sure. It is the doctor who has made us sure of our condition and set the horizons of treatment, recovery, life expectancy. We have been medicalized. We are entirely in the doctor's hands.

Another part of the explanation is the fear of catastrophe and lack of communication that characterize the doctor–patient relationship. Patients are predisposed to believe that doctors have the power to solve any problem. Patients neither wish to nor will accept the possibility that doctors are fallible and make errors of judgement. Doctors are in no hurry to disabuse them. One medical student recently recounted some advice given to her last year by an orthopaedic consultant. 'The patients like to think of us as God. It comforts them – it's not our business to make them think otherwise.'

In addition, as the author of the *Doctor's Communication Handbook* states, 'dysfunctional consultations are common in general practice'. Patients are very frightened of their illnesses. They often come into surgeries with preconceptions that are not addressed. They are diagnosed and prescribed or referred for conditions entirely different from those they believed they had, with little explanation. Often they do not take medicines because they do not think their problems have been addressed or that they are being taken seriously.[2]

These characteristics of medicine and the doctor–patient relationship blur the clear cut lines on which accountable relations are built. The complication of the question 'accountability to whom' affects the question 'accountability for what'. Doctors must show they are working efficiently and safely, demonstrating this through medical audit procedures and management devices like job plans. These measure the volume of work they put in and its effect on the quality of patient care. They do not, however, measure the outcomes of that work.[3]

These problems constantly undermine the stability of the health system. Clinical freedom and medical autonomy make it extremely difficult to test the efficiency and effectiveness of doctors' work. If doctors are neither effective nor efficient they are wasting money. This in turn means the hard choices in health care – rationing, closing hospitals, looking at alternative funding methods – are perpetuated and exaggerated, and politicians, voters and patients all begin asking whether the system is worth preserving. If doctors were really held to account, at least there would be a firm foundation from which to make judgements about the rest of the health edifice.

The answer must be to bring in mechanisms to monitor performance. We shall examine one of these, clinical audit – and the difficulty of overcoming blurred lines of accountability – in Chapter 8. In this chapter we shall look at other management initiatives to hold doctors to account. In both cases we shall find there are serious shortcomings to the systems put in place, often due to the ability of doctors to resist them.

General practitioners

Governments past and present are convinced that primary care holds the key to better, more efficient services: good general practice is cost effective and keeps people out of hospital. A 1987 White Paper, *Promoting Better*

Health, sought to apply lessons learned in the hospital sector from the Griffiths reforms to the primary care arena; making bonus payments for reaching targets in certain specified areas and payments for GPs in deprived areas. But the 1990 proposals were the ones which really shook up the system.[4]

The Conservative Government wanted stronger primary care in order to create a more open, accountable system from the bottom up. It started by revisiting the GP contract – to the great annoyance of the BMA. The new contract had been under discussion since the 1987 White Paper. Its main points were:

- strengthened family health services authorities to replace family practitioner committees

- more information for patients on primary care services

- a list of services defining 'good general practice' including triennial health checks and annual ones for over 75s

- higher percentage of capitation in budget up from 45% to 60%.

GPs resented these changes because they saw their workloads going up and their freedom inhibited.

Fundholding

Contractual issues, however, were dwarfed by the scale of the role general practice was being asked to assume in the new model health system. It was intended to move power away from the producers in the health service – the hospitals and hospital staff – to the purchasers and to allow purchasers to take a more robust attitude to hospitals. This was to be the end of the NHS 'consultants' charter'.

In short, the new model GP would fulfil three roles: first, as the consumer's champion, giving guidance through the NHS labyrinth (the 'accountability to whom' question and a key selling point for a Government which was claiming to empower individuals); second, as financial manager, keeping down the costs of the service as a purchaser while maintaining quality of care (the 'accountability for what' issue) and third as political footsoldier, reopening the historical split between the two elements of the profession.

Spurred on by evidence that systems employing primary care 'gatekeepers' were the most efficient – Britain's total health bill at around

6.5% of gross domestic product compared with, say, America's, which had no primary care system to speak of, running at about 13% – the Government saw GPs as the key firstly to quantifying and ultimately to containing demand.[5]

The financial element was to contain costs. In principle, GPs as purchasers, like health authorities, were to be given annual budgets to buy certain services from hospital trusts – generally speaking drugs and 'elective' surgery – like hip operations, for which there were long waiting lists, and high political controversy where the NHS was seen to be at its worst. Fundholding excluded accident and emergency, urgent surgery and expensive treatment costing over £6000. The idea was to have money following the patient but not to ruin fundholders.

The political dimension was critical to the Government's chances of driving the reform package through. Whereas, before, the GP had always been at odds with the view of the spirit of the NHS – essentially that it was a monolithic structure where teamwork and concensus were key values – now he found his independent status fell very much in line with Government thinking. The fundholder would create a dynamic frontier for purchasing – which initially was largely carried out by health authorities – and this was intended to drive the new accountability into the system. Traditionally GPs, although independent, had been at the behest of hospitals and health authorities, responsible neither for commissioning nor providing treatment, and so divorced from the costs of either. Now they were being asked to do and pay for both. The vision of reversing power from hospital to community, consultant to GP, to allow the economic reforms to bite, relied on enlisting the support of the family doctors. But there was an underlying agenda to increase GP accountability in the long term by making them salaried employees.

General practitioners could use the emotive and time-honoured waiting list as gauge of performance by trusts, and as a whip with which to lash ever higher levels out of them. GPs were playing on the high profile of the waiting list in the NHS. Managers who wanted knighthoods got them down. Those who didn't got the sack. They were backed up by central government initiatives on waiting lists themselves and through the Patient's Charter, which sought to bring total times down across the country.

Fundholding also began to wrest control for budgets out of health authority hands – on average each GP who decides to start fundholding sees a reduction of £1 million in the health authority budget.

In the early waves fundholding was limited to larger practices – which needed to have a minimum of 9000 patients to be eligible, in order to broaden the pool of risk, but in 1996 the number was lowered to 5000 for the standard model of fundholding. As we have seen variations on the theme were encouraged by the Government for larger or smaller practices.

Accountability and primary care

The tendency of the scheme to strengthen or weaken accountability has gradually become apparent. Among the successes are the bringing of decision making and care – like physiotherapy – closer to patients on a day-to-day basis. In addition, the shorter waiting times fundholders secured for their patients, attacked so often for introducing two tierism into the service, have often levered standards up so all have benefited.[6]

And, as a study of 28 fundholding practices has recently revealed, fundholders have 'effected rapid savings in their prescribing costs'. This stems from the fact that drugs budgets are cash limited under the scheme in the same way as hospital services. So fundholders face similar incentives to save. But as the study adds the main gains are made early on and may not be kept up later.[7]

Leading fundholders say the tension between the greater freedom in contracting with trusts and the greater discipline needed to run the fund is creating a new and more dynamic health service. Cheshire GP, Dr David Colin-Thomé, a leading fundholding light, claims it has brought the NHS nearer the patient, challenging inappropriate care by consultants, and helping 'the health of the nation instead of the health of the hospital.'[8]

Specifically, he argues that fundholders should make good the gap of understanding between patients and the health service through individual contact, which ensures efficiency, quality and accountability. 'In the quasi market of the NHS ... there is a gap between the purchaser and the person on whose behalf the purchase is being made. This necessitates another condition – that the purchaser has to act in line with the best interest of the patient.' He concludes that the GP has more incentive than a health authority 'to act well on behalf of the patient.'[9]

Dr Rhidian Morris, formerly chairman of the National Association of Fundholding Practices, points to the strengths of the scheme in terms of the leverage it gives him over hospitals. In the old NHS, where hospitals were linked to the health authority, there was no choice over where to send patients. Now there is – at least for some fundholders.

'There is no doubt that we need the district general hospital for some things – emergency care, urgent and quick treatment, diagnosis and advice,' he says. 'But what I do not want is a patient who has been diagnosed and can be treated in my surgery, sitting in an expensive hospital bed, using up my funds.'

Dr Morris explained that there was a range of alternative services available locally, including a cottage hospital, a private nursing home, a council residential home, all of which offered alternatives to Derriford hospital for conditions that did not need to be treated there.

> If I send someone to Derriford for a week, I get a bill of about £850, just for the bed. That would cost me £310 in the nursing home. If the patient does not need acute treatment, why pay the extra?
>
> I can also do some things in my surgery now – again for considerably less than before – physiotherapy, chiropody, counselling, and we have consultants coming to visit us – one does an obstetrics clinic in the surgery, for example.
>
> This is all better for the patient as well. We often hear about people who are happy with the quality of the treatment they get in a hospital, but find the place impersonal and depressing. We change that.[10]

Fundholding has been and remains the most controversial aspect of the reforms. However, it has not always been the controversy that has bedevilled fundholding. The fear of controversy has led to measures preventing it from achieving its goals.

A report by the Audit Commission painted a varied picture of the scheme and how well it had worked. Many of the criticisms of the scheme pointed to problems with the nuts and bolts of how the management systems worked. 'The majority of fundholding practices do not appear to be especially good at management and networking or achieving a large number of benefits for patients,' it reported. Accountability suffered.

Practices, like Dr Colin-Thomé's, which were 'turning the world upside down', were few and far between, with many practices hindered by limited ambition of what the scheme could achieve for them. There were some benefits, like a reduction in waiting lists, increased efficiency in prescribing, a wider range of referral, but many weaknesses were identified. In broad terms these relate to the failure of the internal market to operate as had been planned. As we saw in the last chapter choice was the fulcrum of accountability and change in the new system. It was intended to set the system on its head – to allow the patient to have power to choose GPs, GPs to have power to choose hospitals and so on.[11] We have seen that choice was extremely limited between hospitals. The same applied to the choice of GPs by patients – as we saw in the Consumers Association report.

The flip-side of the ascendancy of 'choice' was the suppression of 'voice' throughout the system. While, as we saw in the last chapter, this was a clear theoretical consequence of reform and was formalized in crude ways such as removing local authority members form health authority boards, it became a practical part of everyday life in the NHS at the grass roots, among fundholders. So while choice was failing to introduce accountability and change, there was no compensatory mechanism for public involvement that would allow patients to speak up for themselves. As 'voice' was squeezed out, 'choice' – the dynamic which was supposed to empower consumers – was being effectively undermined by market management. The system has become less accountable than ever before.

This problem is explicitly addressed by the Audit Commission report. Patients were rarely consulted in plans for what services they would purchase. Communication with patients was cursory – few even had newsletters. There was little collaboration with trusts or with health authorities to improve services and provide them with a better fit to the local needs of their populations. Contracts were often poorly managed. Few systems had been set up to judge the fundholders' purchasing decisions. The outcomes of treatments were not monitored regularly.

The value for money of the scheme as a whole was also questioned. By the end of 1994–95 fundholding practices had received a total of £232 million to cover staff, equipment and management costs. The report baldly commented: 'The £206 million efficiency savings made by fundholders over the same period, which the regulations allow them to retain and spend for the further benefit of their patients, do not match these costs.'

Clearly the selling point of accountability to the patient is undermined by these criticisms. Fundholders seem unable or unwilling to represent the patient's interests.

According to Anna Coote of the Institute of Public Policy Research, fundholders are falling short of the accountability to patients required of them by the framework set up under the reforms. Fundholders are accountable to the NHS Executive, which requires them to publish documents about management of their funds, to involve patients in service planning and to have appropriate complaints procedures in place. But she points out that only 3% of practices had patient groups, and argues that the mystery of medicine puts the public off.[12]

Leading GPs responded by questioning the appropriateness of fundholding as a dominant mode for general practice. The NHS Executive made clear that it wanted to see a list of definitions of good practice, including the ability to manage a budget. The Audit Commission proposed an accreditation system. One leading GP on the Commission, Dr Tony Mathie, suggested stronger monitoring by health authorities to check on fundholders after two years. Others pointed to the need for 'purchasing tests'.[13]

This is a pressure recognized by fundholders themselves, some of whom are not happy with the increased rationing choices they are expected to make. They are not happy with the exposure of the 'accountability to whom' and the 'accountability for what' questions which traditionally had been hidden. Having more services in the surgery and having the power to choose which hospital to refer to is one thing, but explicitly taking more decisions about who is going to receive the treatment they need and who is not, is causing deep concern.

Dr Christopher Westwood, a GP on the outskirts of Plymouth, became a fundholder in 1991. He was in the first wave, one of the trailblazers of the reforms. In 1996, he left the scheme, saying he refused to make rationing decisions that had traditionally been made at higher health authority level:

> I am not prepared to sit in my surgery and tell someone that there is not enough money in my budget to give them the treatment they need. Those decisions used to be taken by the health authority. That allowed me to make my decisions according to whether or not treatment was needed on a clinical basis, not a financial one. Fundholding has changed that and it could have a very damaging effect on the relationship between doctor and patient.[14]

Dr Westwood's complaints are a particular case of a more general feeling of malaise in general practice. Many GPs feel they have been loaded down with greater responsibility and work than before for not much reward.

The Government has plans to replace fundholding with locality commissioning. This evolution has emerged around the country as doctors have reacted to weaknesses of the scheme that are examined in the next chapter. There is some evidence that commissioning groups may be more open than fundholders to 'voice' and in turn better at expressing influence in this way themselves, particularly where they are dealing with powerful providers. But there is little sense as yet of a fundamental opening up to patient 'voice' brought about by commissioning.

Consultants

Consultants have traditionally been the elite of the system, having worked 20 years or more to achieve their posts, and they have resisted being made accountable to anyone. There are currently some 55 000 doctors working in hospitals in England and Wales. Most work in general surgery and general medicine, obstetrics, gynaecology, anaesthetics and paediatrics.

The number of consultants has risen every year since the reforms were initiated in 1983. In NHS hospitals in England and Wales in 1993 there were 17 560 consultants, 4118 senior registrars, 6803 registrars and 12 851 senior house officers. In public health there were 125 directors of public health, 366 consultants, 388 senior registrars and registrars, 27 senior house officers, and the total general practice workforce was 30 310 – a total of 72 552.[15] Interestingly, every year the number of hospital consultants has risen while the number on the community 'Cinderella' sector has sometimes fallen. Still, there are too few.

The reforms and consultants

Griffiths

Up until the 1983 Griffiths Report, the key duty of administrators had been seen to be to back up doctors. Innovations like the 1974 consensus management initiative sought to resolve tensions by allowing each important interest group a say at the decision making table. But it failed.

Throughout the reforms of the 1980s the Government fused two ways of thinking about commerce and industry – the big and the small. The big, represented by Griffiths, looked at making large institutions, like Sainsbury's or the NHS, more responsive to consumers, with strong accountability, control over spending and a good image. The small focused on the power, influence and virtue of markets over the anti-competitive and professionally dominated monoliths like the NHS. It was largely the first that concerned Griffiths.

He only hinted at the second, but he laid the ground rules for the introduction of change. By introducing principles of what has been called rational management, as opposed to traditional management, which looks to those who have 'made it up through the ranks' to take management responsibility, the report started a progression towards a more 'rational' health system. Griffiths levelled the playing field. However, it was left to the later reformers to paint the lines on the pitch and divide the players into two teams.

Box 4.1: The manager

One of the key figures in the reforms is the former chief executive of the NHS Executive, Sir Duncan Nichol, who worked closely with Kenneth Clarke as he was implementing the measures. In Nichol's view: 'The hidden agenda of the Government reforms in the 1980s and 1990s was to break the power of the doctors. One way of doing this was to set them off against each other. It may not have been explicit at the time, but I think it was certainly an underlying strategy.'

Before the reforms of the early 1980s, he said:

Management had very circumspect relations with consultants – you had to get on with each other to make things work. The order of the day was administration not management – the administrators were there to help the medical staff and to provide whatever they needed to do their job.

There was no sense of 'let's start with what we think the population needs'. The way of thinking was 'what we do around here is this because this is what interests the doctors'. The emphasis was far more on what the institution itself aspired to become – a renal centre or cardiac centre or whatever, and it was important to build up the status of the hospital in that way.

Nichol says:

It is true that hospitals had very old fashioned management structures. Within hospitals there were power cliques. This was the era of bed allocations to specialities, and one speciality did not presume to impose itself on the bed space of another. In this way doctors could build up their own fiefdoms within hospitals.

It was to break down this powerful grip that the general management reforms of Sir Roy Griffiths were introduced. Sir Duncan Nichol says:

Griffiths brought in the notion that managing a system like the NHS was about the same principles as managing any other system: you had to measure the system's costs, its volumes and the quality of the product it was putting out. The NHS had no way of measuring any of them.

The old situation, where money had nothing to do with doctors, where their position *vis à vis* management was to make it clear what they needed to do their work and the role of the administrator was to make sure that it was provided, had to change. There had to be ways to hold the real spenders to account.'

The response to Griffiths was mixed. Sir Duncan Nichol says: 'Of course the clinicians saw this as an erosion of their clinical freedoms. I argued there was not going to be a situation where managers said to doctors you have to treat in this or that way. But there was certainly a battle.[16] And in the words of another analyst: 'it is not surprising that the reaction to Griffiths from the established NHS professions was cautious and predominantly negative. Power was being taken from [them] and a new authority imposed on a well established and entrenched pattern of vested interests.'[17] For Sir Duncan Nichol the key to the new management culture was that managers had some distance between themselves and doctors.

> One of the reasons that it is now easier to manage doctors is that managers are no longer sleeping in the same bed as the doctors. Now there are purchasing organisations – health authorities or GP fundholders, and they don't have to have a day to day relationship with doctors.
> So, whereas before, a hospital manager would not dare infringe on the clinical decisions a doctor was making, the situation is now very different. A manager in a hospital can say, you can no longer do this operation in this way because the purchaser will not pay for it. And you can also say to them why are your colleagues doing twice as many operations as you, why are you behind on using minimally invasive techniques through endoscopes, etc. All of this can be attributed to purchasers, so there is a much greater leverage for management.[18]

Nevertheless, for some managers Griffiths was the beginning of a whole new era. Robert Naylor, Chief Executive of Birmingham Heartlands Hospital Trust reflects on the change general management brought about.

> Griffiths was the main event. Before that we had consensus management, which meant you had a management committee with the hospital administrator, the top financial officer, half of the senior consultants, the senior nursing staff. Everything had to be agreed by everyone – from investment in new equipment to new consultant posts. If you could not get agreement it got referred up to district health authority level, then up to the region.
> The situation was ridiculous, but it changed with general management. It was a major change, and the main thing was accountability – for the first time you knew who was in charge and who was accountable for decisions.[19]

1990 reforms

The two teams, of course were to be the purchasers and the providers, ushered by the 1990 NHS and Community Care Act. The split between the two was the foundation of the internal market, the force that was to attempt to drive competition into the service in the 1990s.

Power was to be devolved as far as possible – further than before. Central arrangements were to be beefed up: a new policy board chaired by the Secretary of State was to give direction where the Griffiths bodies had failed and the service was to get its own chief executive, heading up a new NHS Executive. Regional and district health authority membership was to be streamlined.

It was at the local level that the most radical changes were to be brought in. Trusts were to become self-governing, independent of health authorities, with the power to set pay and conditions for their staff, run by boards of governors and generating income through contracts with health authorities.

Trust hospitals were given more control over doctors. They were able to determine the pay and conditions of medical staff themselves. They could draw up job descriptions. Clinical autonomy on merit awards – traditionally the preserve of doctors since Bevan accepted Lord Moran's contribution to the 1948 compromise – was shattered with the appointment of managers to the committees deciding them. Level C awards – the bottom rung – had a management element added for the first time and, to sharpen up the performance regime ineffectively introduced earlier in the decade, doctors were to be required to carry out a medical audit of the services they provided.[20]

In theory, management control over consultants spread with each annual wave of trusts. From a fraught beginning, in which 57 hospitals took on trust status against a background of scarcely concealed warfare between clinical colleagues, the pace quickened, until by the end of 1995 nearly all of Britain's 500-or-so teaching and district general hospitals had trust status. Implementation of the measures was put off course by medical lobbying and bargaining at a national level and by limited co-operation at local level but the cultural landscape had changed and managers had more ammunition at their disposal. The shifting balance created its own problems. The sense of isolation from the change was bound to lead to some recalcitrance and obstruction from doctors.

Box 4.2: Conflict

In addition to being a medically qualified doctor Jenny Simpson is a hospital medical director and the chairwoman of the British Association of Medical Managers. She is a prolific writer on medical management and one of her most interesting articles is *Managing the relationship between doctors and managers*.

In that piece, Simpson outlines key and obvious principles for effective relationships in hospitals – that they exist to care for sick people; that their driving force is clinical teams; that services are designed around patients; that decisions are taken openly and rationally and with the consideration of the clinical perspective. Power within the hospital, who wields it, where it is located, is another fundamental question. It cannot be hidden away in the traditional decision making of doctors' firms – it must be in the hands of managers who are accountable, not clinicians who are untrained in management. But the managers must involve clinicians too and allow them to run things where they are able to do so.

Ideally, the balance between management and clinical control leads to a stable and happy working environment. In some hospitals, however, there is a 'nightmare scenario', where doctors are only given token input into management, making suggestions which are ignored by middle and senior managers, where real decisions are taken only by managers and where the doctors eventually become demoralized and cynical.

Simpson says that general management has made a difference but that it has had to be tempered with an understanding of the medical profession. 'I would say there are good relations and systems in about 50% of hospitals. The only way management is going to work is if you get doctors involved. It helps if you have got a chief executive who fundamentally respects the clinical process. Important information, for example, on costs, used to be collected in hospitals but it was never made available to those who needed it. Discussion used to take place behind closed doors and doctors had no interest in how much things cost. That all changed with resource management in 1986. That is when clinical directorates started to monitor and control the budgets going through the clinical system. That is also when doctors got involved in the management process.'

Robert Naylor, Chief Executive of Birmingham Heartlands Hospital, 750 bed second-wave Trust, explains that the Griffiths Report increased tensions between him and doctors, but that the establishment of clinical directorates in 1986 helped forge a link between management and profession which saw them through a rocky period leading through the decision to become a trust. 'There was an enormous tension between me and the consultants immediately in the mid-1980s, in the period after Griffiths. I came to the hospital when there was a £200 000 deficit. This and the allocations we were getting were limiting the extent to which we could expand. There was a stand off between the hospital and the health authority – we needed more money and they were not going to give it to us. For me the crucial decision was whether to put the consultants' view to the health authority or the authority's to the consultants. It came down to taking sides and I quickly realised that unless I had the consultants with me the hospital could not work on a day to day basis'.

Interviews with Jenny Simpson, July 1996 and Robert Naylor, July 1996.

The effects of reform

Pay

But despite the spread of managers and the management culture, the doctors still had power *en masse* to influence their pay and conditions both in public and private sectors. Pay scales have remained effectively national. Doctors' salary scales are reviewed annually by the Review Body on Doctors and Dentists Remuneration (RBDDR), established in 1971, which recommends levels of pay for doctors to the Government. There is a minimum rate, with four scales rising above it – in 1993 from £39 475 to £49 580. Merit awards – from £9935 to £47 200, come on top of this – their number and rate decided by the RBDDR.

Fees

There is a lack of clarity in consultants' charges, a point made by the Monopolies and Mergers Commission (MMC). A 1994 MMC report noted 'considerable concern about the lack of transparency of many consultants' charges' pointing to two aspects: giving the patient information about how much treatment will cost before an operation and supply of bills, and second supplying decent information to GPs.

Indeed, according to the MMC, the BMA was powerful enough to create a monopolistic price control system in 1989, with a list of charges for procedures that operated like a tariff, which private operators would have to pay. The BMA fee scale emerged as a response to the attempts by the private insurance industry to maintain margins as medical costs rose in the 1980s. To do this they did not increase the maximum they would pay to a consultant carrying out treatment for three years up to 1985. As a response to this, the BMA published its own list of fees, which it distributed to consultants. In the view of the MMC, this was an attempt both by the BMA and consultants who followed the BMA to keep prices artificially high and constituted a monopoly of the medical profession. It reported:

> With regard to consultants who follow the BMA guidelines, we have identified a fact which operates and may be expected to operate against the public interest, by reason of the particular effect adverse to the

public interest that the following of the guidelines enables the consultants to charge fees for private medical services higher than they would otherwise have been.

It made the same statement for the BMA itself.

The effect this had on relative private and public sector fees for consultants was striking. The MMC said: 'The implied hourly rates of consultants in private practice are generally much higher than those implied in the NHS.' Median gross earnings of consultants in private practice in 1992 varied from £195 per hour for orthopaedic surgeons to £60 for psychiatrists, according to the MMC. By contrast, it calculated that a consultant with a part time contract and a C level merit award at the top of the pay scale, would be paid £25 per hour in the NHS.[21]

Contracts

Consultants' contracts formalize a best-of-both worlds arrangement. Consultants are permitted to work in both state and private sectors and have contracts that explicitly allow for this. Contracts are based on 'notional half days', sessions of about three hours of which there are 11 in a week. There are three types of contract: whole time, maximum part time and part time. Whole time contracts are for a full 11 notional half days a week, maximum part time for ten elevenths and part time for between one and ten. The advantage of the maximum part time contract is that it allows unlimited private practice outside the ten elevenths of the contract devoted to the NHS, whereas whole time allows private practice only up to the value of one tenth of NHS earnings. Those on maximum part time contracts also keep 10% of their earnings, whereas those on part time contracts keep only the proportion that they work. In both whole time and maximum part time contracts doctors are required to devote 'substantially the whole' of their professional time to NHS duties. This, as we shall see, is a source of concern and suspicion. A total of 15 411 consultants held a maximum part time contract in 1992; 1947 had part time contracts of less than ten notional half days.[22]

In their contractual status, as in so many other spheres of their professional lives, therefore, hospital doctors, particularly consultants, had security and autonomy within the NHS and the opportunity of wealth outside it. The settlement was underpinned by the consensus that had prevailed since the formation of the service. This has not fundamentally been changed by any of the reforms.

Time

Consultants have considerable discretion over the arrangement of their time in the NHS. Doctors can tailor their individual commitments within the framework of their half-day defined contracts. Someone who has a part time contract may be justified in working only four or five sessions a week in the NHS. Those on maximum part time and whole time contracts have to spend their ten or 11 half days in the NHS.

These sessions are not all used in the operating theatre, in the case of surgeons. Much time is used up in outpatient clinics, and other 'soft' sessions are used for teaching, study leave and so on, as well as those put aside for private work. The use of sessions has never been rigorously defined, so there is latitude between hospitals, between specialties and between individuals.

Theatre sessions are spent performing 'lists' of operations. There is huge variation between the amount of work surgeons do. There are major differences – those in ophthalmology carry out an average of 508 operations each year per 'firm', the traditional work group of doctors, at an average of 2.6 per week, whereas those in general surgery and urology carried out 1046 at an average of 4.8. The figures are influenced by the amount of theatre time – general surgery is likely to have more 'slots' than other specialties. It is also affected by 'case mix' – the differing complexity of operations that determines the length of time spent on them. In the specialties in the study – ophthalmology, trauma and ortho-paedics, ear nose and throat and general surgery – this varied from between 53 minutes and one hour 26 minutes.

The study went on to use figures for the specialties to examine the difference in activity by district across the country. It found that beneath the average figures there was considerable variability in operating activity. It concluded: 'This means that some surgeons may spend less than 5 hours per week operating in the NHS and others will spend more than 15 hours.'[23]

The pattern was confirmed by the Audit Commission and Monopolies and Mergers Commission reports into hospital doctors. The Audit Commission allowed for the fact that doctors in some specialties have greater emergency and on-call commitments than others, and that some surgical specialties had low operating commitments and high outpatient activity. However, it concluded 'There is a twofold variation in the *average* number of fixed sessions per consultant for similar sized departments with similar ranges of work.'[24]

Private practice

The latitude built into consultants' working conditions has always more-or-less guaranteed them access to lucrative private sector work from the days of Bevan onwards – indeed this was specifically part of the deal. The majority of consultants hold whole time or maximum part time contracts. They are allowed to work one session in the private sector. In the case of whole time contracts, where 11 sessions must be spent in NHS practice, private work must be fitted into the early mornings and evenings. For maximum part timers private work can be done in one session a week, but any more must again be done either early in the morning or late in the evening.[25] As we have just seen, the pressure of work early in the morning can spill over into NHS time. But how typical is this?

John Yates concluded that those surgeons who worked in the private sector carried out an average of two operations per week in the private sector during the working day, and spent between one and four sessions a week in private rooms consultations. He wrote:

> The conclusion must be that most British surgeons are spending between one and three half days a week in the private sector. There is a wide range of behaviour, with some surgeons spending no time at all in the private sector during normal working hours, whilst at the other extreme some could be devoting as much as half the working week to private sector activity.[23]

Other studies have found similar trends. Laing's study for the Norwich Union found that 72% of private sector operations were carried out on weekdays after 9am and before 5pm. He also found that doctors spend varying amounts of time on their private work.

The incentives to practise in the private sector are large and have grown larger. The same study found: 'The earnings potential of consultants as a group has increased substantially as a result of the growth in the volume of private practice.' It went on to compare consultant earnings with other professions, finding: 'Consultants who supplement their NHS income with part time practice generate a total income that makes them one of the more highly paid professional groups in the UK, though they are substantially below the top of the income distribution. A comfortable living, therefore, seems dependent on private practice.'

Supervision

Underlying much of the difficulty with bringing doctors to account are the training and day-to-day working methods in hospitals. Within hospitals doctors work in 'firms'. A consultant will lead this team of doctors, and he will see it as his unit. It will comprise doctors drawn from junior grades who will accompany 'the boss' on his ward rounds, help in outpatient clinics and in theatre.

These difficulties were supposed to have been addressed in measures brought in under the 1990 reforms, which intended to increase control over consultants. Every consultant is supposed to agree a job plan with the trust chief executive, detailing theatre sessions, outpatient appointments and soft sessions. According to the Department of Health the use of job plans is directly linked to the need for greater control with efficient use of resources. A consultant must stick by a job plan, 'otherwise the use of health service resources would be adversely affected'.[26]

However, the Audit Commission found that only 25% of consultants in a survey of 70 hospitals had job plans, 60% of job plans had been reviewed within the last 12 months, but that those reviews often consisted only of an invitation to consultants to review their own plans.

The Audit Commission found job descriptions determining who does what in a hospital to be inadequate. 'Over 40% of the junior doctors surveyed ... did not have job descriptions. Many of the doctors who did have them said they did not cover important aspects of their work.' It also found that in many cases junior doctors were being asked to do inappropriate tasks. The Audit Commission added that the system of clinical directorates was often not working:

> Clinical directorates were to have been the main mechanism for managing staff and activity, but in practice they are often only mechanisms for managing budgets. Clinical directors do not have managerial authority over the consultants in their directorates nor over the junior doctors. The perception of consultants as autonomous and juniors as 'belonging' to them continues in many hospitals.

Finance

Despite the shortcomings, both of the internal market noted in Chapter 3 and the lack of accountability in hospitals noted here, hospitals have made progress thanks to the reforms. A recent study analysed activity data from NHS trusts before and after reform. It found that competition between providers did not significantly reduce costs. However, it did find that 'costs decreased significantly' when hospitals converted to trust status and took on the new management structures and incentives noted in this chapter.[27] It also found productivity increased but that gains were significant only in the first year or two.

Feeling for a way forward

There has been progress in reform despite the limits to accountability. There has been a shift in the balance of power in the NHS away from the providers towards purchasers. Providers have become more accountable, but these changes have been qualified to a large degree by the maintenance and inflexibility of traditional practices in hospitals. The theoretical shift in power is one thing; its successful exercise is quite another and evidence that purchasers have made a substantial difference to high profile and entrenched providers is equivocal.

At the bottom of these questions lurks a familiar dilemma: 'what do we want from the doctor?' Fundholding and managerialism wrapped together two conflicting strands of medicine: the altruistic, individual impulses and ethics of the doctor, who feels a strong duty to the patient, and the wider, utilitarian principles of the greatest good for the greatest number, mixed with concepts of equity and justice that confront strategists and managers. The importance of the latter was greatly emphasized in the reforms.

The other question is 'What do we want our health system to be?' If we can say: 'uncomprehensive, unfair, costly and paid for at the point of delivery' then we save ourselves a dilemma but we also admit the NHS is nothing but an illusion, a cynical wheeze to make the public love their politicians. If we say 'comprehensive, fair, free to those who can't afford it', we are back to asking 'is this financially possible?' It may be, but the doctor may have to change for it to be so. The doctor must become accountable.

Labour

Labour policy is defined often by what it is against – such as the internal market. It attacks GP fundholding for creating bureaucracy and encouraging cream skimming and a two tier service and for the problems it causes with financial incentives obstructing the doctor–patient relationship. These forces may create incentives to think first about budgets and not patients, but the issue is not addressed by Labour in a way that could lead specifically to the resolution of the accountability question. The manifesto states:

> GPs and nurses will take the lead in combining together locally to plan local health services more efficiently for all the patients in their area. This will enable all GPs in an area to bring their combined strength to bear upon individual hospitals to secure higher standards of patient provision. In making this change we will build on the existing collaborative schemes which already serve 14 million people.

This reaffirms the Government's commitment to the principle of GP commissioning and the purchaser/provider split. But it is possible this policy will weaken the accountability of GPs to their populations unless rigorous and energetic attempts are made to uphold it. The White Paper suggests this will be so but we must reserve judgement. As Alan Maynard points out, such structures erode the clear cut financial incentives for GPs to bring consultants to account within the system. However, defenders of commissioning argue it exerts greater purchasing leverage and can keep links with communities open (*see* Box 4.3).[28]

Labour also criticizes the extra-contractual referral system – which exists to allow GPs to refer to health authorities outside formal contracts – as it creates bureaucracy. In addition it criticizes the short-term contract, preferring long-term arrangements. On top of this it says it will return to GPs the right of freedom of referral. On the face of it these policy aims seem contradictory. Moreover, having both long-term contracts and freedom of referral is likely to cause another grey area. What is the role of the GP in either situation? Is the commissioning GP likely to be able to maintain the tension of accountability in a system with large primary care groups and long-term service agreements?[29]

Box 4.3: Locality commissioning

Michael Dixon is a GP in Collumpton, Devon and describes himself as being 'extremely' anti-fundholding. He is now one of 60 GPs in 15 practices that have arranged themselves into four locality commissioning groups beneath their local health authority.

Dixon believes that the market never actually worked the way it was intended. His commissioning group has, however, been able to improve services dramatically by the threat of using the market rather than actually changing contracts around. 'We have been fairly ferocious towards our local trust,' he says, 'But we have not changed a single contract, we have just had that threat backing us up. The quality has improved dramatically – waiting times came down – although the health authority is now short of money which means they have gone up again. 'There are a number of organizational benefits – communication with hospitals and doctors has been speeded up, availability of consultants has improved, outpatient appointments have been brought forward and the procedures have been speeded up. In short the hospital is now listening instead of saying this is the service we want to provide and here it is.'

'We did this without being fundholders, and I think it will be the way forward. I believe the Government is likely to introduce a system where commissioning is devolved to locality teams which will interact with the health authority. The groups would have devolved budgets with which they would commission care and this would maintain clear accountability for funds. The groups would also introduce clearer accountability structures to allow patients and populations to have a greater say in what care was commissioned, and how.'

Interview with Michael Dixon, August 1997.

The impact of wider GP commissioning on accountability, both of the GP to the patient and of the hospital doctor to the GP, is unclear. The 1997 White Paper makes clear that health authorities will have a monitoring role which will hold both primary care groups and NHS trusts to account over their health improvement programmes. This may make the lines of accountability clearer in theory but whether HAs will be able to monitor complex agreements will depend on the form they take.

In opposition, Labour said it would make health authorities more accountable to local populations by appointing non-executive directors from the community to serve on boards. One of the key priorities must be to monitor the work of GPs in commissioning groups and to ensure accountability to patients as well as to the health authority is enforced. It also wants to involve patients in deciding health care agreements to ensure they are consulted by health authorities (under a new Patient's Charter). This will need persistence: as we saw, fundholders had ignored this requirement of the fundholding programme. Alongside this, Labour wants to beef up the Patient's Charter and community health councils as 'local health advocates'. Energy must be invested in making sure these institutions establish and maintain an effective monitoring role. They must keep an eye on the commissioning process.

So, it is unclear what effect widespread GP commissioning will have on creating accountability of secondary to primary care.

Labour pledged before the election to introduce a 'range of levers' to bring hospital doctors to account. These included audit, comparative information on effectiveness and quality, setting tough targets to improve service quality, which would include patient satisfaction as a criterion. Some preliminary measures have been introduced. It also wants to raise professional standards involving participation of all staff. As we have seen, the autonomy of doctors allows them to resist change. As we shall see in Chapter 7, measures such as these have been tried as part of creating a more scientific, rational service, and they have all been effectively resisted by doctors. The Government will have its work cut out.

Finally the doctor–patient relationship is mentioned only in passing. If the challenges facing the system are really to be tackled some far more radical thinking on this point is needed. The Government claims that 'for the first time in the history of the NHS the Government will align clinical and financial responsibility to give all professionals who make prescribing and referring decisions the opportunity to make financial decisions in the best interests of their patients'.[30] This is clearly not new – fundholding did the same thing. For primary care, the separation of diagnosis and treatment could go some way to creating a more rational relationship between the individual and the profession while at the same time separating the roles of the GP that have for so long clouded the accountability issue and created perverse financial incentives.

For all doctors, an effort must be made to address the individual/universal question. Abolishing the Hippocratic oath and replacing it with a modern, negotiated and open doctors' charter, setting out duties to individuals, commissioning areas and wider areas, would fall in line with the structural changes that have been occurring in recent years.

References

1 Heath I (1995) *The Mystery of General Practice.* Nuffield Provincial Hospitals Trust, London.

2 Tate P (1997) *The Doctor's Communication Handbook.* (2nd ed.) Radcliffe Medical Press, Oxford.

3 For a review of clinical audit see National Audit Office (1995) *Clinical Audit in England.* HMSO, London.

4 Secretaries of State for Social Services, Wales, Northern Ireland and Scotland (1987) *Promoting Better Health* (Cmnd 249). HMSO, London; Secretaries of State

for Social Services, Wales, Northern Ireland and Scotland (1989) *Working for Patients* (Cmnd 555). HMSO, London; Secretary of State for Health (1996) *The National Health Service: a service with ambitions* (Cmnd 3425). HMSO, London; Secretary of State for Health (1996) *Primary Care: delivering the future* (Cmnd 3512). HMSO, London.

5 OECD (1996) *Health Data*. OECD, Paris.

6 Timmins N (1997) Labour's unhealthy prescription. *Financial Times*. July 19.

7 Baines D, Tolley K and Whyres A (1997) *Prescribing, Budgets and Fundholding in General Practice*. Office of Health Economics, London.

8 Colin-Thomé D (1996) Speech at Health Service Journal/Glaxo Wellcome debate on primary care. *Health Service Journal*: May 30, pp. 8–9.

9 Colin-Thomé D (1997) *Why Fundholding Should Stay*. Social Market Foundation, London.

10 Interview with Dr Rhidian Morris, May 1996.

11 Audit Commission (1996) *What the Doctor Ordered: a study of GP fundholders in England and Wales*. HMSO, London.

12 Coote A (1997) The democratic deficit, in M Marinker (ed.) *Sense and Sensibility in Health Care*. BMJ Publishing Group, London.

13 Little S (1996) Do fundholders need to pass a purchasing test? *Fundholding*. June 5, pp. 23–5.

14 Interview with Dr Christopher Westwood, September 1996.

15 Wilson R and Allen P (1993) Medical and dental staffing prospects in the NHS in England and Wales. *Health Trends*, **26**: 70–9.

16 Interview with Sir Duncan Nichol, October 1996.

17 Cox D (1992) Crisis and opportunity in health services management, in R Loveridge and K Mayhew (eds) *Continuity and Crisis in the NHS*. OUP, Oxford.

18 Interview with Sir Duncan Nichol, November 1996.

19 Interview with Robert Naylor, July 1996.

20 Secretary of State for Health (1989) *Working for Patients* (Cmnd 555). HMSO, London.

21 Monopolies and Mergers Commission (1994) *Private Medical Services* (Cmnd 2452). HMSO, London.

22 DoH (1979) *Department of Health Briefing*. PM(79)11.

23 Yates J (1995) *Private Eye, Heart and Hip*. Institute of Health Services Management, London.

24 Audit Commission (1985) *The Doctor's Tale: the work of hospital doctors in England and Wales*. HMSO, London; Audit Commission (1986) *The Doctor's Tale Continued: the audits of hospital medical staffing*. HMSO, London.

25 Laing W (1992) *UK Private Specialist Fees: is the price right?* Norwich Union, London.

26 DoH (1990) *Consultants' Contracts and Job Plans*. HC(90)16.

27 Soderlund N, Csaba I, Gray A *et al.* (1997) Impact of the NHS reforms on English hospital productivity: an analysis of the first three years. *BMJ*, **315**: 1126–9.

28 Interview with Alan Maynard, September 1997.

29 Labour Party (1996) *Renewing the NHS*. Labour Party, London; Labour Party (1997) *New Labour: because Britain deserves better* (Election manifesto). Labour Party, London.
30 Secretary of State for Health (1997) *The New NHS* (Cmnd 3807). HMSO, London.

5 Accountable to the public?

When Britain's modern health system was established after the Second World War people were used to queuing and willing to queue and wait for services and treatments, as they had to for food. Now they demand more. In response to the greater expectations of a public used to double-quick service in the high street and shopping centre, the public services have been overhauled. Consumerism arrived in the health service in 1991, with the current reforms and the Citizen's Charter.

But has your ability to determine the kind of health services on offer really changed for the better, as government and management claim? Or ought the new system, sold as more flexible and consumer friendly, in fact be perceived as the result of a clever cost-cutting exercise that has distanced the public from determining how its system is to be run?

Can you hold the system to account for its actions? You may be told that under the reformed service you have more power because you and the doctors looking after you have more choice over how you are treated and whom you are treated by. Is this true? And even if it is, do you think it is as effective a way of getting what you want out of the service as having a proper say in its running?

Politics and public accountability

The Welfare State in general, and the NHS in particular, were explicitly designed as the weapons to fight a specific problem at a particular time – the insecurity caused by free markets in the 1930s.[1] The basic principle of a tax-funded service has been questioned by politicians, doctors and managers alike, but it has remained because it has retained overwhelming public support despite equivocation over the amount of tax individuals are willing to pay.

For politicians the conundrum has been how to court patients and public alike within the framework of their own ideologies. Since the early days of the service, economic and public financing pressure has created a need for a series of reforms, which has had to focus on using management to make delivery more efficient rather than changing the tax funding structure that has underpinned the legitimacy and equity of the system, maintaining at least superficially the principle of equal care for equal need. This has had implications for the accountability of the service to the public.

For three decades after Bevan famously stated he wanted to hear the echo of every dropped bedpan echoing around Whitehall, the NHS ran as a centralized bureaucracy in which patients had little say. In the view of those who created it after the War, it could be no other way. Centralization was part of the NHS.

The finest exposition of this was made by Enoch Powell in his book *Medicine and Politics*.[2] In Powell's view decisions about the allocations of taxpayers' money should always be made by elected politicians accountable to voters. He believed that the financing of health care through the treasury completely recast the fundamental principles of health provision. In a famous and often-quoted phrase, he summed up what this meant for the man in charge: 'The unnerving discovery every Minister makes at or near the outset of his term of office is that the only subject he is ever destined to discuss with the medical profession is money.' Powell went on to argue that because money was now provided by a centralized and distant apparatus, the medical profession saw a 'vested interest in denigration', arguing that the service was poor, shoddy, dangerous, and therefore needed more funds the whole time. It was the politician who had to decide whether or not to agree.

On this point Powell believed strongly that the layman – the politician – should be in charge setting the boundaries. From the top Powell believed a specialist service like health care needed a 'fresh mind', thus a Minister who was not a doctor. This apart, he said, doctors themselves could not run the service because in the very act of running it they ceased to be doctors and became administrators. He wrote: 'In the last resort, all final decision is lay, whether the decision be that of an individual to undergo an operation or of parliament to institute a national health service.'

But he did not leave it there. Powell could not be personally responsible for the thousands of individual clinical decisions taken in the system every week. Powell made the distinction that politicians are concerned with general consequences of individual decisions. Doctors are concerned with the consequences on their individual relationships with the patient of the general decision made by the politician.

The structure of the service should carry the instructions of the Minister into the day-to-day practice of hospitals. As the service was centrally funded, control had always to lead back to the centre regardless of the structural independence of the regional hospital boards. Powell believed, that 'budgetary control is of the essence in all management. It is pursuing the will-o'-the-wisp to look for ways of giving financial independence to the agencies of a nation-wide service.' Nevertheless, he had identified the considerable strain that could be put on relationships by the tension between centre and periphery.

Philosophically, Powell was a believer in the sovereignty of Parliament. He had faith that Ministers, checked by politicians at Westminster, could exercise sufficient control over the system to represent the interests of patients and taxpayers within it. By 1974, however, ministers saw a need to represent the public and the patient in the system, introducing the community health council (CHC) as a complaints measure, and allowing elected local council members on to health authorities. The effect of these moves was to bring public and patient representation into the system, but also increasingly to politicize it.

Reform and public accountability

It is probably impossible to find any single word that could characterize the series of reforms that have been initiated since 1979. But, paradoxically – given the resistance of the profession and, as we shall see, the decline in local influences on the system – one that has been used in justification has been accountability. Starting at the minutest level of the service, with doctors and their clinical freedom, the reforms attempted to replace autonomy with accountability. From there had been built a system of authority with clear lines of authority and accountability, which replaced the confusion introduced in the 1974 reorganization of 'maximum delegation downwards, maximum accountability upwards'. By introducing first management targets then an internal market the performance of a trust or health authority could be judged. If it was not up to scratch, jobs would be lost.

This was a new kind of accountability, however, and it was one that many still feel does not sit well in a welfare system. It was the accountability of the marketplace, of efficiency, of being able to shop around. It was accountability, enforced by the ability to leave a commercial relationship, over the accountability of voice – having a say in what the doctor provides and how.[3]

As we have seen in Hirschman's classic description, exit allows users to stop using the particular service, or move their custom elsewhere within the system. In the case of health this could mean moving GP, or 'exiting' to the private sector – it was the choice factor. 'Voice', on the other hand relies on direct communication between the user and the organization, either through complaint or, if the channels exist, by having a hand in the strategy-making process for the organization.

Choice over voice

In the last two chapters we have followed the theoretical arguments setting the internal market on a new foundation of choice from the patient upwards which was to recast the system. We have also seen how, in practice, the market was limited both by its own structural failings and by the actions of politicians who limited the extent of market outcomes. Within this context, choice was limited too – the accountability that choice was intended to have levered into the system was stillborn.

The story does not finish there, however. The converse of the argument that choice was to provide a new accountability in the system was that 'voice' became increasingly sidelined. In this chapter, therefore, the question is, what happened to patient voice after 1974, when CHCs were established?

The answer, although it may not entirely have been planned this way, was that it was silenced. What pluralism existed in the system before the reforms of the 1980s and 1990s was being undermined. The Griffiths system was unambiguously centralizing, creating lines of management accountable direct to Whitehall and Westminster.[4]

However, the placing of Griffiths' managerial 'moles' in the system, with their loyalties focused towards the Government machine that gave them their jobs, did not work in the way the system's architects had planned. What happened instead was a confused game of tug-of-war, as the managers found their loyalties torn between their operational units and the centre. As Simon Jenkins notes, even political screening to select chairmen for regional and district health authorities could not convince those who accepted what were widely seen at the time to be poisoned chalices of managing the doctors that their loyalties pointed towards Westminster rather than the medical staff. Jenkins writes:

> They took seriously their role in bringing a lay view to bear on clinical priorities, but in practice they were at the mercy of their professional and managerial staffs. Chairmen ... felt themselves caught between the Whitehall devil and the medical deep blue sea. Most opted for the sea.[5]

The failure of the Griffiths measures to deliver the goods, largely thanks to the weak hand dealt to managers and the lack of information they had to do their measuring job with, meant more radical changes next time around – changes that, according to their implementors, would devolve greater power in return for greater accountability.

The claim to be increasing devolution of power to trusts and health authorities was hollow. Jenkins states that Thatcher may have wanted money to be injected into the NHS through the GP fundholder, and for it then to follow the patient around the system. But on the other hand Government wanted greater control over spending in the health service, a desire made stronger by the failings of Griffiths to create real control through the confused instruments of increased managerial power and accountability of politically appointed managers to their masters.

The new health bodies created in the 1990 reforms were staffed along the same lines, only this time some 4000 appointments were to be made. The politicization of management continued. As Andrew Marr points out, this was an overtly political exercise, designed to strengthen political control over the 'devolved' local health authorities and trusts.[6]

In addition to strengthening lines of accountability to the centre, the local bodies had their links to the community cut off. No longer were local authority members appointed to boards of health authorities. In addition trusts did not have to open their doors to the public during important meetings. Health bodies are in effect quangos, unaccountable and obscure locally, watched with hawkish eyes from above. One analyst says: 'while more and more decisions are taken at local levels, vestiges of local accountability ... have been swept away in the NHS reforms.'[7]

Boards of local health authorities are currently made up of five executive directors from the health authority alongside five non-executive directors and a non-executive chair. The non-executive directors are appointed for four years. They are accountable through the NHS Executive to Ministers, and thence to the public. There is no direct link to local communities, whose priorities and agenda may be different from those of the Minister.

Although the role of community health councils was expanded under the reforms to work on purchasing strategies and Patient's Charter objectives they have no representation rights on health authority or trust boards. They have very few staff and their performance varies. More clarity over their role and more funding is required to make them effective.[7]

Anna Coote points out that trusts have unaccountable boards in the same way as health authorities and 'despise' the CHCs as weak. Trusts' communication with the public is patchy and often shrouded behind a spurious 'commercial confidentiality' learned from operation within the internal market. 'This militates against public involvement and open decision making', she writes.

There has been some movement in terms of monitoring the appointment of people to these bodies with the establishment last year of a commissioner for public appointments, but it is again a top-down and remote initiative.

The scrutiny of the system from the centre was increased with the 1996 reorganization, again disguised under the slogan of devolution. With the abandonment of the regional health authorities came their replacement by the National Health Service Executive regional offices. These offices would outline the operation of health authorities in their areas, they would pass on ministerial policy to the health bodies and would oversee the administration of trusts in their areas. Takeovers or mergers of trusts, for example, would be overseen by the executive.

Jenkins writes: 'Ministers run the NHS, answerable to parliament and subject to the most short term of pressures: the generosity of the Treasury each year, the state of the party in the opinion polls and the political vulnerability of the minister him or herself.' Enoch Powell would have argued that accountability ought to be channelled through the Minister in Parliament. In strict terms this satisfies the duty of Parliament to oversee the expenditure of public funds and the administration of systems spending them.

Others argue this is not acceptable. A greater degree of local accountability is needed in those who administer the service to those for whom they administer it. As a result one study states: 'Local health authorities are not accountable to their local populations, but only at a national level: to the Secretary of State for Health and thence to Parliament. The convention of ministerial responsibility to parliament, while theoretically respectable, fails to deliver democratic accountability.'[8] The complexity of public service and the weakness of the systems of accountability – the scrutiny of the parliamentary committee system and the referral of individual cases to the ombudsman – is no force for accountability. These developments are of concern, particularly at a time when health authorities, GP fundholders and commissioning groups are charged with the explicit responsibility of planning services for their areas, leading to ethical and financial dilemmas over rationing services and resource allocation.

Some have argued that to reintroduce accountability, at the very least, boards of authorities and trusts should be opened up again. Beyond this, CHCs could be updated beyond the change in roles that accompanied the 1990 changes, giving them a wider role in monitoring the strategic decisions of purchasers. Rights could be applied to CHCs in the same way as they are to individuals – to monitor, inspect and to be consulted by health authorities.

Local authorities could be brought in to take over local purchasing, allowing democracy to be introduced to the commissioning process as well as bringing together the divergent branches of health and social care under one umbrella. Within a national framework for purchasing priorities this could satisfy local need and demand without sacrificing national equity. Scotland's lead in piloting projects could be followed, with local councils charged with producing integrated social and health care plans and commissioning care.[8] Local authority commissioning would also increase the possibility of integrating social and health care planning with other policy areas such as education, transport and the environment.

Some object that: 'There is little evidence that elected local authorities have engaged in the kind of debate and dialogue about priorities that ... should characterise the NHS.' Instead, a regulatory role is argued for local authorities.[9]

These questions come to the very heart of the issue facing local decision makers – is it possible to involve the public, and if so why should they be involved any more than experts? Accountability is important, and the issues of 'voice' complementing 'choice' are too.

Above all, policy has to be credible. This leads one analyst to suggest that, although user involvement is likely to increase in the NHS and the private health sector, it will do so slowly. In addition, the increase in user involvement will lead to an increasing politicization of the service. Lobby groups may hijack rationing debates arguing for more spending for their particular group, but not taking responsibility for a realistic assessment of where cuts in other parts of the service can come.[10] So 'users' must be balanced by the public at large – since these two groups will have different views on what is spent on health.

Nevertheless, even if there is the power to choose – and this is disputable – there are serious questions as to whether this is an adequate replacement for the public having access to a say in the running of the system locally. In Simon Jenkins's words: 'Citizenship is not a matter of exercising consumer choice of products and services where permitted, and voting once every four or five years.'[5]

The Patient's Charter

Over the top of the structural market reforms predicated on choice and 'exit' was grafted the theme of rights. These came in the form of the Patient's Charter, which set targets for the kind of care and the speed with which that care should be available. It set out seven established rights – access to care on the basis of clinical need, registration with a GP, access to emergency care, referral to a consultant, informed consent to treatment, access to medical records, voluntary participation in training or research – and three new ones – detailed information on local services including waiting times, guaranteed admission date for treatment within two years, to have all complaints investigated and a prompt reply.[11]

The Patient's Charter was used as a shorthand signal by the Government to the voters preparing for the 1992 election that the NHS really was being run for them, and that it was being enshrined in a set of principles, delivered through every letterbox in the land. It received no extra money, however, and was given a cool reception because the targets were seen as unambitious.

The notion of 'top down' reform is seen as a major weakness of the Patient's Charter. A spokesman for the Patients Association says:

> The Patient's Charter represented the beginning of consumerism in the NHS, and in that sense it is the single most important development of the reforms. Fundholding has brought services closer to the patient. But it is the Patient's Charter that has brought more focus on giving them what they need, as opposed to telling them what they want and what they need. But it is very top down, and very prescriptive.'[12]

According to a consumer survey, the Charter is ineffective.

> Only one in four patients could name a Charter right or standard. We put Charter standards in the list of priorities for a good service. And we quizzed patients about how their actual experience matched the charter ideal. Two things were clear: the Charter doesn't reflect patient's real priorities, and the improvements it has laid down aren't being met.[13]

The same report mirrors the Patients Association's concerns. It showed that 'patients would draw up a very different Charter'. Charter standards – single sex wards, food, waiting times – were well down the list of priorities, with other concerns like more communication with medical staff and treatment of pain higher. The survey showed that standards were not being met – a third of patients said the information on the risks and benefits of treatment should have been better, a third said they did not know their nurse by name and 26% said they weren't given enough information on discharge.

Chris Ham suggests that league tables introduced under the charter mean that there is greater information in the public domain, and points to independent research showing dissatisfaction with the NHS is falling. On the other hand he states that a report by the Ombudsman in 1994 was critical of the NHS's performance in responding to complaints.[14]

Public consultation

In the absence of direct representation on health bodies, the Government has claimed that patients can exercise their voice throughout the contracting process. As Ranade and Appleby point out, the Government's reforms have attempted to build the patient's view of the quality of health services into the commissioning and contracting processes. In Ranade's words: 'The contracting process ... provides an excellent vehicle for negotiating explicit quality standards and targets.' The ideal situation, she continues, is where GPs and purchasers are in consultation with user groups as one of the criteria for drawing up their purchasing priorities, which has implications for allocating resources to particular groups. These are incorporated into the purchasing authority's 'statement of purpose', which looks over the medium term at the types of services it is to offer to meet the specific needs of patients and users in its area.

Thus the concept of user 'voice' should be incorporated into the contract-based commissioning process. Ranade and Appleby point to 'considerable activity on this front', with district health authorities in close consultation with GPs over patient input to the process of commissioning.[11] The Local Voices initiative, launched in 1992, is an attempt to boost this kind of activity.[15]

Redmayne, in her latest survey of purchasing authorities, notes health authorities placing greater emphasis on publicizing plans through measures such as road shows, local free papers and public meetings. However, she notes that it is not clear how effective these measures are in reaching their audiences, or how or whether the information they gather is put to use in the purchasing plans. Focus groups, 'have your say' days, surgeries, public surveys and tear-off strips in purchasing plans are all methods used.[16]

Some authorities target specific groups with their material. North-West Anglia Health Authority has developed a 'healthy horizons' policy, with a briefing pack to 'those who have said that they wish to be involved in shaping future services for children and families'. According to the briefing, workshops are held to assess what people value in the service they use, provide or purchase, particular issues or people in specific areas of the region, and priorities for action development and change. Along with the health authority, the county's housing and education departments are involved – a sign that local and health authorities may be working together.[17]

But how effective are these participatory mechanisms? According to the Institute for Public Policy Research (IPPR): 'In practice, Local Voices initiatives have been used to consult the public, rather than to enable them to participate actively in decisions.' This suggests that assessing whether and how services have changed is a much more difficult process than starting initiatives.[8]

As Redmayne and the IPPR have noted, the integration of patient views into consultation processes in the context of commissioning services is patchy. In another study on rationing, Redmayne and two colleagues indicate problems surrounding setting the right questions for the right circumstances. There are difficulties of 'which public is being consulted?' Different areas may have different priorities but so may groups within the same area. The authors conclude that case studies they carried out 'suggest that the results of such consultation exercises are used to legitimate strategies already being followed rather than leading to any changes'. It also suggests that the public is not as keen to be consulted as either the Department of Health or health authorities suggest.[9]

Another study on rationing illuminates a further problem: the relationship between public opinion and other ethical considerations. The author writes: 'Priorities chosen by the public do not necessarily offer the most equitable solutions in relation to the original aspiration of the NHS of equal treatment for equal need.' The research found that the public's decisions were not 'value free'. They tend to favour treatment for a younger rather than an older population, and attitudes to those who had contributed to their own ill health – for example smokers – indicated a preference for resources to be directed elsewhere. So different groups of people have different priorities in the rationing arena.[18]

Public consultation within the current system seems limited in the information it can deliver and by the 'acceptability' of the results it turns out. As has been noted elsewhere, the public may not be prepared to take decisions, they may be guided by phraseology of questions or express 'unacceptable' preferences. Taking this one step further, it could be argued that the whole attempt at public consultation – illustrated by the difficulties surrounding rationing – is an exercise in self-delusion. This is a view set out by David Hunter who believes that the difficulties in interpreting the public's views, and of dealing with prejudices against, say, AIDS patients, 'present real challenges' to the health authorities, who have 'feverishly been commissioning, conducting and analysing public opinion surveys'. He asks: 'Of the many voices of the public, who should managers be listening to?' He believes the path of least self-delusion is that of 'muddling through elegantly'.[19]

Citizens' juries

Others argue there are processes that, when linked with the structures noted earlier at national level and within health authorities, trusts and GP surgeries, could help to illuminate the current non-debate and improve the quality of decision making by being clearer about what is being decided. They attempt to address the fact that although decisions are difficult and the processes seem difficult to formulate, the questions have reached a level of importance and profile that can no longer allow them to lie. One of these processes is called a citizen's jury.

Citizens' juries present an interesting attempt to seek legitimacy and to focus public thought on issues. They invoke the principle behind legal juries, that a group of ordinary lay people can and ought to be capable of coming to decisions on complex sets of facts, making objective judgements based on their interpretation of them, which can be held to represent judgements of the 'common man'.

In one interpretation, the citizen's jury can be used to overcome a passivity in citizens caused by the centralization of power by governments, and their definition as customers choosing between services on offer rather than determining what those services should be – in short encouraging them to raise their voice. Juries themselves can play a part in reinvigorating the atrophied democratic forms that at present characterize the British system. Citizens' juries can 'help to build a habit of democracy', and can be applied to health planning, education, environmental issues and taxation policy.[20]

A citizens' jury in Cambridge and Huntingdon dealt with the question of rationing services, and indicated the immense challenges faced by the public dealing with complex ethical and economic issues. The 15-strong jury was presented with a number of witnesses ranging from the Director of Public Health, to cardiologists and senior members of Royal Colleges, who presented information on the details of particular treatments alongside arguments for and against national priority setting. There were clear limitations to the process. Attitudes to doctors constrained the jury's legitimacy in the jurors' own minds. Their conclusions were limited – 15 out of 16 agreed there should be public consultation on priority setting, but 14 out of 16 said there should be guidelines, offering flexibility, rather than binding statements on specific treatments. Despite the difficulties, the Director of Public Health, Dr Ron Zimmern, himself involved in the Child B case, was impressed, saying it helped with the process and could be a useful part of the process of priority setting. But Dr Zimmern does not believe he should be forced to take into account what juries say.[21]

Citizens' juries have been used in other areas. One in Walsall, near Birmingham, for example, looked at the provision of palliative care for the terminally ill in the town. The basic concept underlying discussions was providing the best service for the community within a budget of £600 000 set aside by the health authority. That service was to provide 'quality dying'.

Combining financial considerations with such sensitive issues was a challenge for the 16 jurors, who included a student, a pianist, a sales manager, a housewife and a builder, but they believed that it was important for members of the community to have a say in what decision was taken. One, a schools inspector said: 'The local people have got to have a say. After all it is our families, who are going to be dying. We need to be involved.'[22]

A total of four options for arranging palliative care services was put to the jury. The first was care at home, which the jurors thought was a right patients should have, but could not be the basis for services for the whole community. Family members could find the caring too stressful, and it was thought home care would be best provided alongside other options. In any case, family members or carers should be given support and information.

The second option was for a hospice, which appealed to many jurors because there was a lack of facilities in Walsall and patients often had to travel outside the area to receive care in the right setting. But some felt that hospices were not liked by patients who thought that they were being 'written off' by being sent there. They also had financial concerns – the £600 000 budget would not cover the costs, and the health authority or local hospice appeal appeared unwilling or unable to raise funds.

The idea of a special ward in the local district general hospital was originally seen as attractive, but the popularity of the option receded through the four sessions and in the end only three jurors supported it as a single option. It was agreed, however, that there was an urgent need to improve palliative care in Walsall anyway. The nursing home, option four, was almost a non-runner to start with, with no support. In the end, however, the jurors were attracted to the idea that a nursing home with specialist palliative care facilities could be offered – a nursing home with a difference, in the words of one GP who addressed the sessions – which could combine the hospice and nursing home models. Funding could attract the private and voluntary sectors – already active in providing nursing homes and hospice facilities – to form a partnership, perhaps, with health authority involvement as well.

The sessions were addressed by a member of a voluntary cancer group, the community health council, Walsall's Director of Public Health, the health authority chief executive as well as medical staff from hospitals and the community. The reaction of jurors to the sessions was interesting. A sales manager said at the beginning:

My view is that the health authority has already made up its mind and wants us to agree. It's pretty clear from what he said that the chief executive does not want a hospice because it is too expensive, and is steering us towards a combination of the other three options. If we don't they won't listen.[22]

However, Michael Evans, the health authority chief executive said: 'The whole point of this exercise is to have a debate, and there is no chance of doing that if I come along with ideas that I am not willing to change.' He said he had put the arguments for the four options in the context of the money that was available to spend on them. 'I was very impressed with the level of debate in the sessions. Several of the jurors showed a keen interest and asked me questions that showed they were getting to grips with some difficult issues.'[22]

Mr Evans, unlike Dr Zimmern, said he thought it was important to take the jury's decisions seriously and to publish the authority's reasons for not acting on them if that was the decision taken. After the exercise the health authority published a document, in which it outlined a strategy stemming from the sessions, and commented: 'The health authority appreciates the quality of the report. The jury was faced with some of the same challenges and constraints as the health authority and has responded with a realistic assessment of future policy. The recommendations appear to be broadly acceptable to the authority.' Parts of the strategy involved increasing the £600 000 put aside for palliative care, more nursing support and adding a consultant post and increasing the information available to patients. On the 'hospice with a difference' it says: 'We believe that it would be realistic, and true to the wishes of the jury, to develop a strategy which describes the evolution of the "hospice with a difference" into a full hospice over a period of years.'[23]

Exercises such as this are expensive – £16 000 a time, a point both Dr Zimmern and Mr Evans made. Nevertheless, in Mr Evans's words: 'It was a useful exercise, and something we would consider using to examine difficult questions once every few years.'

It is easy to dismiss citizens' juries and other consultation exercises as expensive, particularly if they are not seen to deliver high quality decisions. Some argue that a budget for these practices – limited to a proportion of total spending in the same way as clinical services have budgets set – would help legitimize the procedure itself.[10] Many believe there needs to be greater public involvement in decision making at local levels in the health system, particularly as the decisions – like rationing –

are becoming more explicit, more concentrated into definable decision making groups and more focused on specific communities.

Nevertheless citizens' juries are open to another criticism of public consultation that if they were used as a wider forum they would be hijacked by the pressure group.

Pressure groups

If democratic forms of voice contribution and accountability were promoted, one consequence would be to increase the politicization of the system. This would reopen it at a local level to a phenomenon that has increased greatly at a national level – the pressure group. Ham notes that consumer groups have historically been less well organized than producer groups because they have had less of an input into policy making at the highest level. Yet it is widely recognized that the voice of the user in the service – whether we call them patients, consumers or citizens – has become more powerful and groups promoting it more widespread.[24]

With increased awareness of specific diseases and the options for treatment, patients have organized themselves into groups to exert political pressure through the system at Westminster. Alongside this they are busy putting out information on their specific treatments to their members.

The activities of these groups have become sophisticated, and the complex issues in the health service are grasped and understood from the patient's view. In one publication, the National Cancer Alliance sought views from cancer patients about using the NHS. The NCA used focus groups comprising 75 patients in four areas of England, trying to draw participants 'from a range of different sources' – and therefore legitimacy for the study. They were asked to think about cancer services in four categories – information and support, approach of health professionals, speed and time to think and the environment and location of services.

Patients wanted as much information as possible when they needed it, according to the survey, but most found the service did not meet these needs. One patient recalls being told: 'You don't know what you don't know.' Some made it clear they expected to have to make difficult decisions based on the information, but also stated they believed it was up to them to make them. 'I'd like a bit of honesty about the treatment, what it involves and how successful it is', said one. 'There's quality of life ... I'd rather have five good years than ten miserable ones. I'd like more information so that I could decide and I'll take responsibility for that if I snuff it in five years.'

The survey notes: 'Participants reported that they frequently had difficulty relating to health professionals, and had been unable to develop an effective working relationship with them.' There were examples of kindness and sensitivity. There were also examples of the opposite. One patient said: 'It was a case of "I'm very sorry, it's malignant, here's a date for the operation, here's the door." '

They called for as much information as possible. Doctors should improve their communication skills, there should be easier access to second opinions, a 'linkworker' to guide patients through the system would be useful, and GPs should be brought into the local cancer system better. In addition they called for a 'generally pleasant environment' in hospitals, with good transport links. Early hospital appointments should be available, and diagnostic procedures should be speeded up.[25]

The fundamental question about the NCA and the hundreds of other pressure groups crowding into the health arena is 'whom do they represent?' What legitimacy do they have? The NHS has always worked through a system of bargaining for status, money and conditions of work by pressure groups working within it.[26] However, the consumerization of health care has led to greater 'bargaining' from the outside. As Peter Riddell points out, their prevalence is a function of public disillusionment with national politics and political parties. In the case of the NHS this is compounded by the lack of access to debate and the mechanics of the system at local and regional levels. This may lead to the pressure group exaggerating its claims in order to get its voice across, generally asking for more and more money. We are back to Powell's cacophony. But as Riddell also observed:

> It is the role of politicians and parliament to mediate between competing interests, expressed through campaigns by pressure groups or otherwise. Politicians' complaints about the media attention that pressure groups receive, and the time they have to give to them reflect their own failures and the lack of respect in which parliament and the political class is held.[27]

Blocking off the dialogue that legitimate forms of public participation encouraged is likely to add to the erosion of this respect.

These pressure groups, then, can be seen as a response to the blocking of other forms of voice accountability in the NHS. In the absence of formalized and credible channels of influence, patients have to shout loud to be heard over the buzz of the market. Whether they are heard or not, and whether they should be, are matters for contention.

What is clear, however, is that they are creating the noise. The stridency of their criticisms is very much in the tradition of what Powell recognized as the 'vested interest in denigration' caused by centralization of management and financing. The volume with which this is carried out by the pressure groups amplifies the sense of crisis at the heart of the system. Allied to concerns raised by finance-induced reform, these could, over the longer term, undermine faith in and erode support for the NHS. Indeed, surveys paint an increasingly gloomy portrait of public faith in the NHS. One, in December 1997, found four out of five were pessimistic about its future.[28]

Box 5.1: From patient to pressure group campaigner

For some patients illness becomes a journey of discovery. Through that journey, the patient has to adjust to an entirely different life. Life itself may be shorter, living it may be more difficult and understanding how to survive while dependent on drugs or other treatment requires complete re-orientation. Some patients see this as a challenge and learn all they can about their condition. In some cases, they go on to start disease specific campaigns, promoting the cause of fellow sufferers and making claims on public money for their disease. They have completed the journey from uninformed patient to knowledgeable activist and challenge the medical establishment. The question is, do they fulfil a valuable function, and does their ability to speak give them a legitimacy?

Becky Miles, Chairwoman and founder of the National Cancer Alliance gives an interesting account of her conversion. In 1987, when she was expecting her third child, she became ill. She was diagnosed as suffering from sarcoidosis, a condition where lumps appear around the lymph nodes.

She says: 'I had a long period of therapy treatment with steroid drugs. I very soon decided that doctors could not read, and so I started to read everything I could about sarcoidosis. They opened me up and said that it was non-malignant. The person who did that was a general surgeon. It did not seem to be non-malignant to me, and so I went back. I was seen by another doctor, a thoracic physician, who said the pathology in the previous test was not done properly. In 1990, I went to the Royal Marsden Hospital in London. By this time I was extremely ill with a compressed vena cava and in retrospect I had only days left to live. I was re-diagnosed, this time with Hodgkin's Lymphoma – a cancer of the lymphatic tissue. I could not believe it. It seemed to me that the doctors did not know anything, and that I needed to get into the driving seat. My attitude was to learn everything I could about Hodgkin's disease and haematology.'

Becky goes on to say that once she had been properly diagnosed she went on to chemotherapy and received 'superb treatment'. But it was the trouble that she had to go to to ensure she got the proper treatment that worried and frightened her.

She says: 'To get there I had to go through a total of 13 different consultants. Why do people called doctors behave so badly to each other and to me? But there are still choices and nobody made me aware of this at the time. For example they were constrained by a drugs budget.' She explained that when on chemotherapy the person needs anti-emetic drugs to stop vomiting. There were two types: one where hair loss is likely and the other, where there was a chance of losing fertility. Becky says: 'Their crucial decisions were taken with cost-benefit in mind. They start you off on the cheap ones and if they don't work move you on to the more expensive ones. The cheap ones have the fertility problem, but they knew I had two children already. As the first ones did not work, they moved me on to the second and when I asked why they didn't give me those first, they replied: "We knew you had two children already." That is indicative of their attitude. I'd actually rather be bald with a third child. I should have been empowered so I knew about the choices, and the doctor should have informed me about them a good deal better.'

In these circumstances patients are extremely vulnerable and in great need of protection, and need to set up grounds to help themselves.

Interview with Becky Miles, September 1996.

Labour

Consumerism has revolutionized the way social services are viewed. The patient/consumer/citizen/voter is a far more demanding creature than in 1948, but this does not change fundamental pressures – there is still great demand on a limited supply.

What has changed are ways in which society has adapted to the problems. In the past, through structural changes in the system, the 'voice' of patients was enlisted to add accountability to the system – and to instill efficiency into it. More recently 'exit' has been used.

The Government has made it clear that it wants to see greater managerial accountability and openness to the public. It has announced it will open up board meetings of NHS trusts to the public, suggesting that this would indicate to communities that trusts were there to serve them. In addition it said that appointments to boards in 1997 would reflect local communities, patients and GPs and had also asked local authorities to put forward names. It said this would be a first step to opening up appointments procedures.[29] The White Paper added that trusts must publish management information and annual details of performance for use in league tables. These are positive developments.[30]

Labour is committed to a new NHS Charter and establishing new rights and responsibilities – for example everyone should have access to a GP, but should use the GP responsibly. Complaints procedures should be established and monitored under the charter and appointments systems should be personalized to give patients better information about their condition and treatments and to help reduce or at least explain waiting time.[31] This echoes the rights-based approach suggested as a basis for rationing procedures (see Chapter 8). Much depends on what the definition of a 'right' is, and at what level the targets are set. The success of local health advocates again depends on what they set out to do.

As well as trusts, the Government has suggested opening up health authorities to local accountability both through consultation and open meetings. However, it has ruled out guaranteed seats on trusts for local councillors which is seen as a retreat from pre-election commitments to greater local representation on boards.[32] Given that their role as commissioners of health care will be maintained as the Government keeps the purchaser/provider split, this is pressing. It has drawn attention to the draining of accountability through the way responsibilities are divided in the system, but it has stopped short of unifying the commissioning of all care – social as well as health care – in a single agency. On the other hand it is piloting Health Action Zones to try and break down chinese walls.

The information, which the consumer model has been successful in bringing out of the system, can be used not only in contracting, but in measuring the performance of the system and making judgements on it. The public should be enlisted in the quest to do so – and on a wider front than on focus groups such as citizen's juries. If it is accepted that individuals are capable of making competent and rational commercial decisions it should be possible to argue that they can make participatory ones too. In theory at least, they can be competent citizens as well as consumers.

References

1 To trace the development of thinking behind the NHS see British Medical Association (1938) *A General Medical Service for the Nation*. British Medical Association, London; Beveridge W (1942) *Social Insurance and Allied Service*

(Cmnd 6404). HMSO, London; Ministry of Health (1943) *Statement on a National Health Service* (Cmnd 6502). HMSO, London; Ministry of Health (1943) *A National Health Service* (Cmnd 6502). HMSO, London; *National Health Service Act 1946*; Watkin B (1975) *Documents on Health and Social Services: 1834 to the present day.* Methuen, London; Webster C (1988) *The Health Service Since the War: volume I.* HMSO, London; Klein R (1995) *The New Politics of the NHS.* (3rd ed.) Longman, Harlow; Timmins N (1995) *The Five Giants: a biography of the welfare state.* HarperCollins, London.

2 Powell JE (1975) *Medicine and Politics.* (2nd ed.) Pitman Medical, London.

3 Hirschman A (1970) *Exit, Voice and Loyalty: response to decline in firms, organizations and states.* Harvard University Press, Cambridge, MA.

4 Griffiths R (1983) *NHS Management Inquiry.* DHSS, London.

5 Jenkins S (1995) *Accountable to None: the Tory nationalization of Britain.* Hamish Hamilton, London.

6 Marr A (1995) *Ruling Britannia: the failure and future of British democracy.* Michael Joseph, London.

7 Coote A (1997) The democratic deficit, in M Marinke (ed.) *Sense and Sensibility in Health Care.* BMJ Publishing Group, London. For further discussion of the 'democratic deficit', see Wistow G (1993) *Community Care.* Sept 30, p. 20..

8 Cooper L, Coote A, Davies A *et al.* (1995) *Voices Off: tackling the democratic deficit in health.* Institute for Public Policy Research, London.

9 Klein R, Day P and Redmayne S (1996) *Managing Scarcity: priority setting and rationing in the National Health Service.* Open University Press, Buckingham.

10 Perri 6 (1996) *What Future for User Involvement in the NHS 6.* Briefing for Demos Seminar.

11 Secretary of State for Health (1991) *The Patient's Charter.* Department of Health, London. For a good explanation of the Patient's Charter see Ranade W (1994) *A Future for the NHS?* Longman, Harlow.

12 Interview with Patients Association, July 1996.

13 Consumers Association (1995) The NHS: what's the verdict? *Which? Way to Health.* June.

14 Ham C (1997) *Management and Competition in the NHS.* (2nd ed.) Radcliffe Medical Press, Oxford.

15 NHS Management Executive (1992) *Local Voices: the views of local people in purchasing for health.* EL(92)1. NHSME, London.

16 Redmayne S (1996) *Small Steps, Big Goals: purchasing policies in the NHS.* Centre for the Analysis of Social Policy, NAHAT, Birmingham.

17 North West Anglia Health Authority (1995) *Children and Families Healthy Horizons.* NWAHA, Peterborough.

18 Bowling A (1996) Health Care Rationing: the public's debate. *BMJ.* **312**: 670–3.

19 Hunter D (1993) *Rationing Dilemmas in Healthcare.* NAHAT, Birmingham.

20 Stewart J, Kendall E and Coote A (1994) *Citizens' Juries.* Institute for Public Policy Research, London.

21 Quoted in Timmins N (1996) How would you spend the health service budget? *Independent.* May 13.

22 Interview at Walsall Citizens' Jury Session, August 1996. The following material is taken from attendance at the Walsall Citizens' Jury.
23 Evans M (1996) *Walsall Health Authority Report on Citizens' Jury on Palliative Care, September 1996.* IPPR, London; Lenaghan J (1996) *Walsall Citizens' Jury: improving palliative care in Walsall.* IPPR, London.
24 Ham C (1992) *Health Policy in Britain.* (3rd ed.) Macmillan, Basingstoke.
25 National Cancer Alliance (1996) *Patient-centred Cancer Services? What patients say.* National Cancer Alliance, Oxford.
26 Eckstein H (1960) *Pressure Group Politics.* Allen & Unwin, London.
27 Riddell P (1996) Pressure groups, media and government, in Waldegrave W, Secrett C, Bazalgette P *et al.* (ed.) *Pressure Group Politics in Modern Britain.* Social Market Foundation, London.
28 Social Market Foundation (1997) *Ready for Treatment.* SMF, London.
29 DoH (1997) *Board meetings of health authorities to be opened up to the public.* 30 June (press release); Speech by Frank Dobson to Unison Annual Health Group Meeting, 30 June.
30 Secretary of State for Health (1997) *The New NHS* (Cmnd 3807). HMSO, London.
31 Labour Party (1996) *Renewing the NHS.* Labour Party, London; Labour Party (1997) *New Labour: because Britain deserves better* (Election manifesto). Labour Party, London; Harman H (1996) *Cut the Waste, Cut the Waiting.* Labour Party, London.
32 Butler P (1997) Dobson orders purge of 'dead beat' board members. *Health Service Journal.*

6 Replacing fear: funding British health care

When Aneurin Bevan came to write down his thoughts on socialism in 1963, he called the volume *In Place of Fear*. In it he set out his reasons for believing that ensuring health care is available to all who need it regardless of ability to pay was a duty for the country as a whole.[1]

Bevan rehearsed the arguments for a number of alternatives to the tax-funded system that he introduced in 1948. One by one he ruled them out: private insurance, means testing, group insurance, employment-based insurance.

For Bevan 'The essence of a satisfactory health service is that the rich and the poor are treated alike, that poverty is not a disability, and wealth is not advantaged.' The tax system, because it was progressive, was the best way of safeguarding this principle.

The irony of Bevan's creation – which was intended to ensure peace of mind as well as promote health and cure disease – was to be found in the title of his book. So far from replacing fear, the health system he left behind him has caused a good deal of insecurity in politicians, the medical profession and the public ever since its creation. Bevan was, of course, aware of what he had created, and added what amounts to a warning to the end of his reflections. 'What emerges,' he says, 'in the final count, is the massive contribution the British Health Service makes to the equipment of a civilised society. It has now become a part of the texture of our national life. No political party would survive that tried to destroy it.'

Alongside the structural problems in the system were the questions of demand for the services. The system was based on third party payment. The accepted wisdom before the NHS was set up was that it would create a healthier population, which would need less and less medical treatment, and therefore place less of a financial burden on the system as time went by. But the scale of the mistake was apparent within months of the service starting. As Bevan put it himself: 'We never shall have all we need. Expectation will always exceed capacity.'[2]

Limits had to be found, and although the Guillebaud Report stressed the sustainability of the system, it was clear that funding pressure would grow in future. The search for an answer brought politicians face-to-face with the medical accountability issue we noted in Chapter 2.

At first sight the reasons for rises in costs seemed clear: ophthalmics, which had been calculated to cost £1 million, in fact cost £22 million, the dental service £43 million instead of £10 million. Demand, at least for spectacles, dentures and medicine, it seemed, had been severely under-estimated.

But the Guillebaud Committee's report provided a contrasting analysis. In an accompanying paper by Richard Titmuss and Brian Abel-Smith, the contribution of inflation was included for the first time. They found that, after the figures had been adjusted for inflation, the real rise in the cost of the service between 1949–50 and 1953–54, was much lower than the headline figures suggested. In addition, since the economy had grown, health spending had fallen as a proportion of GDP from 3.75% in 1949–50 to 3.25% four years later. The cost per capita of the service had not changed either.[3]

Guillebaud's report was believed by some to have saved the NHS, but it did make clear that the service was only ever likely to be able to provide a proportion of all the health care needed in any year. However, it vastly underestimated the future growth in demand on the service – suggesting spending would increase by 8.1% between 1951–52 and 1971 – an annual increase of 0.4%, which has never been achieved. Indeed, when general inflation is accounted for, the rise is some 3% a year; when medical inflation is included it is just under 2%. It is clear that a signifi-cant rise is the key trend in NHS funding since 1948. As Appleby points out, Titmuss and Abel-Smith underestimated the extent of population ageing and did not account for the increase in technology costs or the fact that the service may have understated demand when they carried out their work. Nevertheless, it added that the belief of both Bevan and Bever-idge before him, that the NHS would diminish demand for its services by creating a healthier population less in need of them, was a fallacy.[4]

But the NHS has become more efficient in its use of this money. Total discharges and deaths – the measure used, until 1990, for hospital activity, rose from 3 million in 1949–50 to 8 million in 1989–90. Acute discharges and deaths per 1000 population nearly doubled and acute discharges and deaths per bed went up 2.5-fold. New outpatient cases have doubled, completed dental courses trebled, prescriptions doubled.

For the politician, in Klein's words:

The dilemma of policy was not how to restrain consumer demands through the price mechanism but how to reconcile the professional imperative of doctors to maximise the treatment given to any one patient with the need to maximise the health of the population at large, between an absolutist ethic of treatment and a utilitarian approach to resource use.

But, as with so much else in the NHS, policy was conducted implicitly. There was little clarity over what happened to funds within the NHS.[5]

Responses to funding pressures

Bevan's observation that the NHS would destroy whoever tried to destroy it has defined the policy arena on NHS funding from 1948. Despite the major pressures for change we noted in Chapters 2 and 3, there has been extraordinary consensus on the issues. The consensus has worked at several levels.

The chief agreement about funding has been reflected in the fact that no significant alteration to the tax-based settlement has been publicly raised. While the consensus at another level – the role of the doctor and manager – has been pulled apart throughout the Conservative supply-side shake up, demand has been untouched.

The NHS has been able to win an average 3% increase in funds per year from the Treasury – although that figure falls by 1% when specific medical inflation is taken into account. In many ways the system has worked well at keeping costs down. Britain's centralized system, with Treasury control, the fact that the NHS is a monopsony purchaser, and the gatekeeper split between primary and secondary care have all worked to keep it sustainable up to now. Funding has been increased incrementally.

However, there is growing concern about the threat of a funding crisis, as we saw in Chapter 1. Indeed some analyses of spending argue that between 1981 and 1991 actual spending has fallen by significant amounts below what economists calculate is needed given demographic and technological pressures. The visible results are that waiting lists grow. But the underlying question is: how much of Britain's health demand are we willing to satisfy? And, in turn, beneath this lies the question: how much of the demand for health is actual medical need? These are value judgements about the nature of illness to which we will return in the next chapter.

Responses to the 'funding gap' argument have been varied – the previous government stated that there was no question that an NHS providing care free at the point of delivery was sustainable because it has been able to increase its efficiency in the past, but it is clear there will be pressures for change and it is possible that these will force the top layer of the consensus to shatter, despite the attempts to preserve it through the recent reforms.

The f-word and political management

In Autumn 1996, senior health services managers warned that the system was running short of money, that there would be overt rationing through the winter, and that the service faced the biggest financial crisis since the catastrophic winter of 1987. The Association of CHCs said the NHS reforms had been introduced to deal with the problem of trusts running out of money at the end of the financial year. It was still happening. In June 1997, the Institute of Health Services Management carried out a survey in which 90% of managers said services in their areas had been subject to rationing because of 'financial pressures'.[6] And by October there were reports that Tony Blair was willing to make an exception to his rigorous public spending ceilings in the case of the NHS, already promised more than £1.2 billion in the budget for 1998–99, to the relief of the DoH which had argued the need for £300 million more to keep waiting lists down in 1997–98. Pressure has been upwards. September 1997's figures for total patients waiting were 1.2 million, up 14% on the previous year. Those waiting over a year rose 47 000 to 57 500 over the previous quarter.[7] In human terms, the five and a half year wait for a hip operation would have officially been 18 months one year before.[a] These were the worst ever figures and looked very bad for a Government elected on a pledge to cut waiting.

The Conservative reform programme was carried out against a background of financial crisis that had its origins in five years of extremely tight budget settlements leading up to 1987. In that year the system came close to breaking down. The highly publicized deaths of two children after cancelled operations led three Royal Colleges to state that hospital services were close to snapping and a total of £270 million emergency funding was injected into the system. In January 1988 Mrs Thatcher unexpectedly announced on the BBC's Panorama that a review of the health service was under way.

The Health Secretary, John Moore, argued that the financial crisis in the health system could be solved by more private finance and provision, encouraged through tax incentives. He also argued for a hypothecated sum of money raised for and spent on the National Health Service. This would clarify the amount taxpayers were putting into the service and break the idea that the NHS was free.

He was opposed by Nigel Lawson, who believed in increased charges, stating that it was absurd that they raised a lower proportion of NHS spending than in the 1950s. Thatcher thrashed out a compromise with

---

[a] National waiting list helpline

Lawson and Moore's successor Kenneth Clarke – those over 60 received tax exemption on private medical insurance.[8]

However, the major changes were to be the supply-side alterations we have noted previously. The Government effectively ducked the twin issues of asking if enough was spent on health and, if not, who should pay the shortfall, reasoning that the answer to these questions would not become clear until the system used the money it received more efficiently. This thinking made up the package of measures in the notoriously sketchy 1989 White Paper, presented by Clarke.[9]

The Government turned away from a radical look at health service financing for political reasons, but was able partially to satisfy three key policy requirements – containing spending, meeting demand and diffusing blame – in what was proposed on the supply side.[10] Budgets were to be rigorously controlled. The efficiency index would dictate that pound for pound NHS trusts would deliver more activity each year, and the autonomy of those groups, vested with powers to act as free agents in the marketplace, would make it easier to diffuse blame – for example over rationing – than it had been with direct management lines from the hospital to Whitehall.

Nevertheless, within a decade, as we have seen, the same questions have returned. Was demand being met? Was enough being spent? The questions about financing have returned.

Alternative sources of finance

Accepted wisdom has it that the public will not brook cuts to services, that it wants them there when it needs them, but it is also not keen on paying more in taxes.

The 1996 British Social Attitudes Survey shows that when people are asked simply whether they want to see more spending on health, 77% of people say yes, ranking it above other services, and that the number has increased since 1991, when it dropped from a 1987 level of 78%. However the survey found that answers on questions of tax contradict answers on spending because most individuals already feel their personal tax burden is high enough, regardless of their income.[11]

Health, however, is a big programme and gains greater support than smaller ones, partly because of the social solidarity it engenders. It may be easier to introduce different sources of finance in smaller programmes – such as higher education, where students must now pay fees. In addition, it is clear that the poorer groups that use the NHS are more in favour of increased spending, and those wealthier households, which have private arrangements, less so. The wealthy still believe a system is needed providing core services, not least because of the unpleasant social consequences to them of having no safety net.

The consequences of these results suggest that the electorate, the taxpayer, the citizen and the user of the service are all unclear about what they want out of it and how their relationship with the service changes in each of these modes. It also suggests that if there were greater clarity about the methods of tax raising and funding, there might be more clarity about what the public would accept in terms of reform.

Until now politics have dictated that the service remained centrally tax funded. It is unlikely that it will remain centrally funded without being a tax-based system. Other centrally provided methods – insurance systems in France and Germany, for example – are not favoured for two reasons. First, the transaction costs of collecting money through a number of insurance funds drives the costs up. Even separating health into a national insurance fund is likely to drive up costs in the UK. Second, as we shall see later, one of the qualities of an income-based tax system is that it redistributes resources from rich to poor, and so reinforces equity. Maintaining a centrally funded system but undermining this principle would make little political or economic sense. The rationale behind Bevan's choice of tax remains.

Charges

There are, however, alternatives, which can and have operated at the margins of the service since it was founded. The first are charges for some elements of the service, which have been in existence since 1952, and over which Bevan himself resigned. Bevan's principles would not allow any dilution of the 'free-at-the-point-of-delivery' basis of the service.

Box 6.1: Comparisons

One 1995 study of six OECD countries – Canada, Germany, The Netherlands, Sweden, USA and Britain – makes it clear that cost sharing is evolving around the world as health systems face up to the threat of demand outpacing resources.

The USA, where State health care is at its lowest level, presented its population with the greatest likelihood of having to bear part of the costs of a particular episode of care above and beyond the entitlements outlined in their particular insurance package. At the time of the survey, for example, US citizens had an average of only 61% of their medical bills met by public funds, whereas British people had 93% – second only to Sweden in the study. In Britain for example, there was (and remains) no co-payment for inpatient or outpatient care and a prescription charge of pharmaceuticals. In Sweden, there was a daily payment for inpatients, and outpatients for the first prescription item and a reduced one for each further item. In Germany there was a payment for the first 12 days of inpatient care with nothing thereafter and no charge for outpatients or payments for drugs.

The American system was the most complex, with three broad categories of payment system running alongside each other. Medicare, the federal system that looks after old people, had three types of co-payment for inpatient care. There were deductibles – where the first $n of the total treatment cost is met by the patient, coinsurance – where the patient pays a set percentage of the total charge, and maximum lifetime benefits, where patients have so much credit throughout their life, after which they must pay the whole cost of any particular treatment. For outpatients, there were deductibles, coinsurance payments and balance billing – where a patient will meet the difference between what a doctor charges and what the scheme sets as a cost ceiling for that particular treatment. For pharmaceuticals there is 100% cost sharing – the patient pays the bill.

The Medicaid system, operated by states for the poor, employed cost sharing systems, but they varied from state to state. In the private sector, which covers the majority of the population whether through employer or personal schemes, there is a wide variety of methods, each varying by insurer. For inpatient care there was coinsurance of 20%, $200 deductibles, balance billings, and maximum lifetime benefits. For outpatients coinsurance was levied at the same rate, co-payments from $5 to $7, deductibles of $200, balance billing and maximum lifetime benefits. For pharmaceuticals there were coinsurance, co-payments deductibles and maximum benefits.

The different strategies load different proportions of risk on to parties to each agreement. So maximum lifetime benefits load the costs at the end of someone's life – when they are most likely to need long-term treatment and perhaps least likely to be able to pay for it. Deductibles on the other hand present a fixed up-front payment. So someone looking for $300 of treatment will get a worse deal than someone looking for $3000. Coinsurance spreads the payments more evenly over the whole cost of treatment. Balance billing gives an incentive to those on schemes to persuade their doctors to charge lower fees. All of these instruments are inducements to people signing policies to consider their position.

In Britain public and total spending on health have diverged – although the divergence was greater in the 1950s and 1960s – which suggests that an increasing bill is being met by co-payments and by people buying care through the private sector. Whereas according to OECD figures in 1980 total spending stood at £13 344 million, with public spending accounting for £11 953 million of that, by 1991, the total figure was £38 000 million, with only £31 670 million met from the public purse.

In Britain the array of cost-sharing methods is limited. Direct cost sharing – where an actual payment for services is made – does not exist for NHS outpatients or inpatients, but there are payments for prescription charges (either each time or as a season ticket), eye tests and dentistry.

There is 'indirect' cost sharing. Pharmacists, for example, can substitute generic medicines for brand names, which brings the costs down. The rate of generic prescribing in Britain increased from 21% in 1982 to 45% in 1992 fuelled by reforms. A selected list scheme also limits the range of medicines that are reimbursable by the NHS – such as analgesics for mild pain, antacids, cold and cough medicines, laxatives and tonics. In the private sector there are many different methods of imposing co-payment regimes.

There are serious difficulties with cost sharing from the standpoint of equity. The classic case against cost sharing is that it is a regressive system – charges at the point of use are weighted against the poor who have to pay out a higher proportion of their incomes to meet them. Approaches to solving this problem founder. First, giving flat-rate exemptions to those who are judged unable to meet the costs of payment can undermine the basis of the system, because they can become so wide that the revenue gained from the charges is negligible. This means increasing the rate of charges, which is always highly politically sensitive and creates a huge leap from the subsidy to the payment. Graded systems, where charges are made on the basis of ability to pay, would be bureaucratic and expensive, although these arguments are perhaps weakening with the advance of technology. In addition, in recession, a greater number of people are likely to become unemployed as the economy stops growing. They will gain exemptions, but it is at precisely this point that the need for income from other sources than tax is at its greatest.[12]

The sensitivity of the issue is made obvious by the Government's unclear position on it. The Government has launched a fundamental review of the system, 'ruling nothing out'. It has said it will not rule out charges for GP visits but maintains, at the same time, that there is no threat to the universality of the system.[13]

Doctors, formerly opposed to charges, may be changing their views as recent polls have shown and research published in December 1997 found only one in three people would be discouraged from visiting their GP if there was a £5 charge.[14]

Tax breaks

The question of tax breaks appears to have been kicked out of play at the moment, with the ending of the rebate for over-60s taking out health insurance.

Hypothecation

One other area that is receiving renewed interest is hypothecation. Arguments over introducing a 'health stamp' have been a constant companion to the NHS.[15] In one analysis, taxes over time have been 'disconnected' – separating the tax bill from the services on offer and obscuring the logic, efficiency and legitimacy of public financing from taxpayers.

Legitimizing the system and allowing taxpayers to understand how their money is being used are not accomplished by the current set up. Hypothecation along with greater democracy are advocated to make the system clearer. The goal should be to give voters a voice over the real level of the NHS budget.[16] This would enhance the legitimacy of public health care.

These arguments have traditionally foundered on treasury power. Arguments against claim that once taxes are hypothecated it is almost impossible to bring them down or control spending. People are more likely to say there is not enough, rather than there is too much. But as has been noted earlier reform up until now has focused on issues of microeconomic efficiency. It has avoided asking the big questions: do we spend enough, are we willing to spend more? Hypothecation would be a way of asking these questions and it could avoid some politically unappetizing extremes to which we now turn.

Moral dilemmas, radical economics

The funding debate has been driven from the extremes. From the right, the British health system is faced by two distinct problems: the moral and the economic. But they are also strongly linked. It is to break the link between the lack of responsibility created by the system and the economic consequences – essentially offering British people an open-ended bank account on the NHS with no questions asked – that proposals are made to end the NHS's supremacy in the health system, replacing it with a private-based one. The controversial starting point is that there is no moral legitimacy for the system and therefore no economic legitimacy.

Right wing analyst David Green says: 'The welfare problem is not primarily financial, but moral. The difficulty is not so much that the welfare state cannot be afforded, but that welfare programmes have tended to impair human character.'

Green and others argue that human nature is at its best when it assumes responsibilities. Responsibility is inherent in the choices made within the market, and while a standard criticism of the market is that it is amoral, the counter argument is that in fact the market is embedded in morality. Green looks back to a golden age:

> Historically, a combination of a state minimum with the additional support of charities and mutual aid associations offered superior protection because it attended not only to cash needs but to character. Support services should appeal to people's strengths, not their weaknesses.

His view is that the Welfare State should be thought of within the context of a voluntary sector, which should be able to receive Government grants if in need but should be encouraged towards a more independent spirit.[17]

Green believes the system is not able to control this demand in any other way than rationing health care because there is no price system that allows people to make their own judgements. To overcome this in his view the private sector has to step into the gap. But these arguments ignore the possibility of greater responsibility through clearer information and more transparent structures outlined in preceding chapters and above.

Politics and privatization

The word 'privatization' has haunted Conservative health secretaries since 1979. In fact, while privatization has undoubtedly been made easier by the reforms, a counter argument that the reforms have saved the service from the need to privatize can be sustained.

It is worth pausing for a second, however, to ask exactly what is meant by the word 'privatization'. The British system has never been the monolithic state system of legend. As we have seen in previous chapters, GPs have jealously guarded and successfully maintained their right to practise as independent contractors, not salaried to the state. Consultants are independent too, although salaried, and are allowed to practice privately during one or more sessions of their contracts – an effective subsidy of the private sector.

Community services have been the 'Cinderella' of the health system – currently they are provided by a mixture of health authorities and local authorities, the one funded through general taxation, the other through local taxation, top up grants from the centre and, increasingly – particularly for long-term care – through private arrangements.

But accusations that the service was being set up for privatization were most strongly focused on the recent round of reforms. GP fundholders were to be able to refer patients to private providers – how long would it be before they could accept patients paying through private medical insurance policies, preferring these to others because they did not affect their budgets either for treatment in the surgery or in hospital after referral?

Hospital trusts were floated off from health authority control, to be given greater powers over what they did with their money, what treatments they provided and from where they took patients. They were to be able to build up pay-bed units to take private patients. They could buy and sell assets and land to generate better returns from capital that had lain dormant since the foundation of the NHS.

It is now a rarity to find an NHS dentist, although there are suggestions of a reinstatement of services for the elderly. Patients are expected to pay for treatment. The provision of dental and ophthalmic services, like the introduction of prescription charges, are not seen as fundamental challenges to the system. They are seen as necessary sacrifices to maintain the public structure of the bulk of the service.

Like the reformed NHS, the private health care system can be divided into two parts: the purchaser and the provider. Demand and supply. When people talk about privatizing the health service, they generally talk of one of these two things.

If tax funding and public sector purchasing were maintained, publicly accountable agencies would still be in charge of the allocation of resources, and would technically be able to hold private sector operators accountable for quality, efficiency and, to a degree, equity, through the contracting system.

More contentious would be allowing private insurers control over public funds because it would be a good deal more difficult to detect and regulate the aspects of market failure that characterize this part of the system – cream skimming and adverse selection.

If the State's role in taxing to provide services is going to shrink to allow greater choice – even at the expense of equity, solidarity and, security – then a system that allowed private control of funds to be spent on private insurance would be acceptable. The political and social issues raised by this, however, appear far greater than they do when thinking in terms of privatizing NHS trusts or transferring them to the voluntary sector. Of course, moving both purchasing and provision into the private sector is one step further still.

The private medical insurer can be either a provident association like BUPA or PPP, or a for-profit organization, either large or small, ranging from a major composite insurer like Legal & General to a cluster of small organizations. The number of subscribers to private medical insurance (PMI) was 3.2 million at the end of 1995 and the total number of people covered by policies was just below 6.2 million.[18]

Looking ahead, the prospects for growth in PMI are not dramatic, according to Laing, with no prospect of a return to the boom years of the 1980, but unless the sense of crisis surrounding the NHS lifts, some growth is likely.

Another area where the private and public sectors are lined up close together is in the Private Finance Initiative (PFI). Here, the Government's objectives are difficult to gauge. The PFI is intended to bring private funds into capital projects in the NHS. Private construction firms and banks come together in consortia to bid for projects. They do not receive money from the Government to complete the buildings: they have to finance the construction themselves. The PFI is intended to make private capital available to the public sector – reducing the Government's borrowing requirement in the process but also to import private sector management techniques.

The first objection is that the cost of private capital is higher than government borrowing. The Government's response has been that the private sector will be able to make efficiency savings that, over the long term, will more than recoup the costs of servicing loans from private banks. Other criticisms follow the same logic as objections to private provision of services: private sector companies running hospital services and seeking efficiency gains. Only a handful of schemes have been agreed so far, but it appears that the Government is committed to the PFI as a key way of raising finance in future. But for the moment clinical services, radiology and pathology will not be included in PFI.

Opting out

Failing to address the financing question has meant that the current relationship between the two sectors is blurred and confusing to the patient. The nature of the split is changing as the reformed NHS looks to become more efficient and to attract business from wherever it can. As private medical insurance is sold on the basis of weaknesses in the NHS, the basis of the reason for buying it is changing and so the private sector has to react. Under these circumstances there is no strategic direction for the private sector. The 'blurred line' defined by time and amenity between the two sectors allows the NHS not to face questions about rationing its services head on. This blurred relationship reflects that no clear cut decisions on who should do what and therefore on rationing public health care provision have been attempted and reflects that a complex and contradictory set of motives defines use of the system which themselves have implications for equity.

One study finds that those people who have private medical insurance are more likely to be dissatisfied with the NHS than those who do not. The same study found that regional variations in waiting lists had a direct impact on regional take-up of private medical insurance. 'In regions with longer waiting lists, long or short-term, there is more individually-purchased private insurance.'[19]

Going beyond this analysis, the authors conclude that those who bought private insurance are less likely to want to support the NHS financially. They identify a spiral that could undermine support for the NHS; any cuts in service could increase private insurance and therefore help to undermine support for the NHS. In addition, those who are likely to leave the NHS are those who are its best advocates – the middle classes.

The converse would be to offer a higher quality of service in the NHS through putting more money in to clear waiting lists or raising the quality of the hotel services. But this would paradoxically have a negative effect on the equity of the service, if one accepts the definition of equity that allows wealthy people to take out private health insurance, leaving the NHS to those who cannot afford private premiums – because it is likely that it would prevent wealthier people from taking out private health insurance, attracting them to the NHS. Any increased spending in the NHS will go to these people, who are likely to be better off. This will make the service more regressive. This is a theme to which we shall return later.

According to Roderick Nye of the Social Market Foundation, a split between public and private sector is crucial. He believes there are several options: a system used by everyone some of the time, as now, or by some people all of the time, as in some continental European systems.

David Green believes the best way is to have a public system that is used by some people all of the time. He advocates a system where consumers make a choice each year to join a care-delivery organization, deciding how much they are willing to pay for what level of care, in the same way as they renew their home insurance policy each year. They receive a rebate from what would have been spent on them in the NHS (about £650 a year), which they can spend and top up on a personal scheme. The payout would reflect age, ranging from 90% for the oldest people to 40% for the under 20s, similar to the principle under which the weighted capitation system works for health authorities now. This would bring a notion of responsibility to people's decisions about health care.[17,20]

Green also advocates a return to the voluntary hospital system of before the war. He argues that such a system would revitalize the provision side of the service and weave the hospital back into the fabric of the community whence it was plucked by nationalization in 1948.

He states that voluntary hospitals were in reasonable health before the Second World War – producing annual surpluses of income to the tune of £100 000. He also points to the hospital contributory schemes that allowed lower income groups to make contributions to their care, with 10 million people covered by 1936.

For people on welfare, a guaranteed health care package would be available – a 'safety net' service that would give access to services as and when they were needed, but which would differ from the services used by other parts of the population, who would be able to top up their packages with extra income from the rebate given by the Treasury. They would also be able to pay lower amounts to cover their health costs than their rebate, giving them discretion to spend the money as they saw fit.

The key to Green's system is that it legitimizes an incentive for underprovision through personal choice. Instead of a service that is all things to all men and that does not allow the public to decide what kind of health package they want to pay for, like the American health maintenance organization (HMO) system it allows each person to decide what level of cover he or she is willing to buy.

A similar approach was taken in a report by National Economic Research Associates (NERA). The NERA paper called for the replacement of the bulk of the NHS as a tax-funded system with a competitive compulsory insurance market.

The study advocates drawing up a guaranteed health care package. Social solidarity would be safeguarded in this way, and the public would have a key role in deciding what was to be included and what excluded from the system. Efficiency would be safeguarded in the system that operated above the safety net because it would be operated by competitive insurance companies, which everyone not covered by the State minimum would be obliged to join.

The NERA prototype system therefore starts with the Guaranteed Health Care Package (GHCP) that will be available to all, regardless of ability to pay. For the population not on benefit, insurance funds will purchase services defined in the GHCP for their members. Everyone must insure with one of these organizations, and insurance funds must accept anyone who applies for coverage. The insurance companies would be free to offer their members services over and above the basic GHCP entitlement. Contracts will determine the quantity, price and quality of services offered by providers – GPs and hospitals – to insurers.

The Government would set up a regulatory and licensing framework. Co-payments would be introduced for the items on the GHCP.

The paper argues there is a GHCP at present in Britain – health authorities and doctors use waiting lists and prioritize treatments to create a *de facto* list of services that are not provided. That list is not, however, defined clearly. Work should start on defining it. The total funding of the health care system should be increased to make up for underfunding of the system as it exists now. A co-payment scheme should be introduced.

Thus the individuals would be able to choose what level of care they wanted to buy into and pay accordingly rather than accepting the rationed offerings of the State.[21]

William Laing points out in his critique of the proposals, that they enhance the ability of individuals to choose, but equally they encourage people to think carefully about what health care they need. He believes this could be used to engineer good practice into the system. He writes: 'As a purchaser of a GCHP in NERA's brave new world, I personally would be happy to choose a no grommets, no tonsillectomy health insurance fund, which contracted with doctors who had agreed to work to research-based best practice protocols and which offered rapid access to effective health care.' In short he accepts there are strong arguments to allow people to opt for a system that provides less than the NHS is currently set up to provide.[22]

There are significant objections. The first is the cost of collection that we have noted above. Second there are cream skimming problems. Would a larger private sector based on rebate promote equity? Would the safety net be of as good quality, efficiency and so on as the private sector? The question of defining a GHCP does mean confronting difficult ethical questions about what health care the State is bound to provide. And lastly there is the question of the acceptability of forcing individuals to make decisions about their health care, given the knowledge deficit.[23]

Green believes individuals must make decisions: 'Struggling with choices is part of the human condition. You can't devise a system that takes that struggle away so that the responsibility for your life and death is somebody else's.'[24]

Professor AJ Culyer suggests simpler funding arrangements: a hypothecation of funds from general tax revenues in the way discussed above. Co-payments would not work because it is the doctor who tends to decide on the treatments, and it is not the doctor who would co-pay. Instead, why not pay the doctor, the system we have with GP fundholders? Also co-payments stop people from using primary care – the part of the system that makes it cost effective by catching problems early and avoiding the need for expensive secondary care at a later stage.

Partnership

In one analysis the supply-side reforms have prolonged a weakness that has accompanied the system since it was founded: that in its constant efforts at reform and change, it can only remain a victim of its own success. It is also argued that the notion of treasury control – used against hypothecation – is a 'myth', and that the real determinant of the proportion of our national income we spend on public services is economic performance.

The author, Professor Nicholas Bosanquet, argues that the ambitious goal of better health for all can no longer be met by the rigid structure of the NHS. It needs a more flexible partnership approach. In Bosanquet's view, this points to the need to define the core of what the NHS is for. A future system could 'Guarantee access to health services for major illnesses and for preventative services, but within a context of increased competition in supply and direct payment for some services.'[25]

The method of meeting demand while maintaining competition in supply can be achieved only by loosening the rigorous grip on spending. Bosanquet sees partnership as a way forward that allows individuals to take control of their circumstances, providing a possible solution that does not inflate demand by making the existing services better and thus stoking it to unmeetable levels. It allows flexibility in looking for solutions, promotes competition among providers and shares the cost of developing services into the future between the taxpayer and the user. One area where the Government is looking at proposals for a partnership scheme is long-term care. Proposals under which individuals either take out an annuity on retirement to cover long-term care costs or pay into a long-term care insurance policy, with incentives to do so were published in 1996 and a Royal Commission is currently examining options.[25]

Long-term care

The use of a partnership scheme has been applied to long-term care – at the sharp end of the demographic time bomb. This is an area where the role of the Department of Health has diminished over time and administration is increasingly led by the Department of Social Security, local government, and social services.

In 1970, for example, there were 77 500 long-stay geriatric beds in the NHS. In 1995 there were 53 600. This is against a background of an ageing population in which the over 85s increased from 472 000 to 1 million, from 0.9% of the population to 1.7%.

At the same time there was an increase in nursing and voluntary home places provided in other sectors from 192 800 to 509 400, most dramatically in private nursing and residential homes.[26]

So it is clear that the capacity for medical care for the elderly has declined and social care has increased, but social care is means tested. Before 1993 the means test was carried out by the Department of Social Security benefit office, but now it is carried out by local authority social services that, along with private providers, have taken over control of social long-term care for the elderly.

Long-term care is financed through a number of sources. First there are the long-term geriatric beds in NHS hospitals, which are provided free like other NHS services. Local authorities are encouraged to spend social service budgets in independent sector residential and nursing homes rather than on their own facilities. In addition a £54–£60 allowance is paid to residents of independent homes, whereas this is not paid to local authority home residents. Local authorities therefore have to make up the difference if they send people to their own homes. Income support is also used as a source of funding, both for those who are on it when they go into care and for those who go into a home on a self-pay basis and subsequently run out of money.

Since the 1993 reforms the most important trend has been the increase in self-paying residents. Some 28% pay for their own long-term care, particularly as capital, including a home, can be taken into account in the payment of fees.[26]

The sources of funding long-term care for the elderly reflect the problems of the 'blurred line' between public and private sectors and make clear that it has always been a grey area. Is it provided by the NHS, or is it not? Is it 'health care' or it is 'social care'? In fact, caring for old people has always fallen between these definitions, and as a result, there is still considerable confusion over what to expect and from whom in later life.

NHS continuing care beds are there to deal with elderly people who are admitted to hospital with medical conditions and who need medical care. If it is judged by medical staff that a condition has been stabilized then people can be discharged, but people often stay in hospital for the last months of their lives. Domiciliary care, where people are able to stay in their own homes with support from community teams, has traditionally existed alongside NHS care. Domiciliary care is often preferred by people who need to be looked after in old age – particularly in comparison to often grim NHS long stay wards. But many fear its role is threatened because of changing family patterns which mean the crucial role of informal carers – family members who can offer help in caring for their aged relatives at home – is being eroded. Families now live further apart, and women are increasingly involved in careers in their 30s, 40s and 50s – the time when they would traditionally have looked after their ageing parents. On top of the growth in the elderly population this is seen by many as another crucial pressure bearing down on the ability of the system to cope with the problems of long-term care.

Current thinking on meeting long-term care costs revolves around insurance and capital protection. Long-term care insurance lies at the centre of the plans, and two schemes were proposed in 1996 that amount to incentives for taking out insurance.[27]

There are also proposals for annuities to cover care costs for people who need it immediately.

Groups representing the elderly such as Age Concern and Help the Aged have deep reservations about such proposals, in that they do not tackle the fundamental problems of long-term care because they do not confront the central issue, which is that the services are going to use more and more money in future.[28] Others say that asset protection has a logic to it, that more people have more capital at the end of their lives now, and therefore are in a better position than before to meet costs. In short individuals are richer in relation to the State than they used to be, and therefore can and should take responsibility for paying for their care.

However Laing believes some unfairnesses need to be addressed. He favours – in common with Age Concern – extending public funding for the nursing element of care. Currently the whole cost of nursing home care is met by the individual, in the same way as residential care is paid for, but nursing is provided free in the NHS, and so there is an argument that it should be free in the long-term care structure. This would make explicit the difference between hotel and care costs in long-term care.[29]

More fundamental proposals are outlined by the IPPR. The IPPR advocates examining social insurance options, which would set up a separate national insurance fund for long-term care to which all taxpayers would contribute throughout working life. These possibilities could be used in tandem with partial equity release schemes where a percentage of equity capital (your home) is used to buy insurance coverage. That proportion of your property reverts to the insurance company when you die. A significant point about these proposals is that they implicitly accept that the private sector is here to stay.[30]

The provision of long-term care illustrates a possible way forward to resolve the pressures of growing demand on services where increasing expenditure is constrained. It also resolves the problems of increasing demand by improving supply. The question is, do people think it is acceptable? Effectively care in old age has been privatized.

Public interest regulation and cost

Many of the objections to privatized systems focus around the vulnerability of the patient. This runs across all insurance products and health, whether permanent health insurance against incapacitating injuries or private medical insurance, there are no exceptions.[31] People may not be aware of excesses in their policies – and although insurance companies claim they should read the small print, the point surely is, that the print needs to be larger if insurance is to play a wider role. Nevertheless, the patient is often unaware of the cost of treatment. A consultant may charge over the benefit maximum provided by an insurer such as BUPA, which the insurer will fail to meet. The difference will not be met by the insurer, and so the patient has to pay. If they don't, they could receive a visit from the doctor's debt collector. Of course, it is again up to the patient to negotiate the price. But this is often neither appreciated, or may be subject to the same problems of small print.

The need for regulation

Last year the Office of Fair Trading (OFT) examined the public interest problems thrown up by private insurance.[32] The report looked at four different kinds of products available through private insurers – private medical insurance, permanent health insurance, critical injury insurance and long-term care insurance. It found that the products on offer across all these groups were complex and often difficult to understand. Consequently it was difficult for consumers to shop around between policies, because they often did not know how to compare them. In addition policy premiums were likely to rise faster than inflation. This was a cause for concern because, for people who had private insurance, the ability to shop around by moving between providers was inhibited by the inability to insure previous conditions. This could lead to being 'locked in' for life with a single insurer. On top of this there were underwriting practices that were considered to be unfair. These practices were known as 'moratoria' underwriting, whereby customers' medical histories are not checked to allow them to take out instant cover.

Private medical insurance (PMI) – the largest sector of the private insurance market – presented specific problems. First, plans were often difficult to understand. A system whereby industry-wide standards are implemented enabling easier comparison is urged by the OFT. One way of doing this is to establish a list of 'core benefits' and 'core exclusions' that consumers could use as a guide for the comparison of policies.

The OFT also made recommendations for other parts of the private insurance market. Permanent health insurance offers approximately 2.5 million people insurance against a disability preventing them from work by guaranteeing their salary. However, moratoria underwriting was criticized, and PHI policies presented an even more difficult problem in defining what was included and not included than in the case of PMI.

All of this suggests that in regulatory terms the private insurance market has some way to go before meeting standards of 'fair trading' that would allow it to operate on a wider scale. A fundamental shift in principles is required: it is not defensible to run a public service on the basis of *caveat emptor*.

Structural changes to the market need to be considered to make the provision of treatments fairer and better. For example, elderly people face much higher insurance premiums because of the need to renew policies annually. Allowing people the chance to insure for the long term is a possibility.

Cost

The report also recommended that the public be made more aware of the likelihood of premiums rising at the outset of their policies. Research by the OFT showed that, in recent years, PMI premiums have risen by between 6% and 12% per year above the retail price index. It says: 'Over the long term, increases at these levels, even allowing for some trading down, appear unsustainable.' The insurers argue that several reasons lie behind the inflation: increased incidence of claims and increased costs. Increased claims were due to GP fundholders steering patients towards the private sector because they could then shift them off their own budgets, eagerness among policy holders to get a return on their premiums and a greater awareness of the medical treatments on offer. Costs were rising, according to the insurers, because of medical technologies, fee rises for specialists and use of more sophisticated diagnostic equipment.

This is a significant objection to increased use of the private sector in meeting national health care needs. The NHS, through the gatekeeper system, has managed to keep costs down. Abandoning this could lead down the American path of high cost, uncomprehensive health care.

The wider use of private insurance products is also likely to be regressive. Analysis by economists at the London School of Economics for the Joseph Rowntree Foundation found that private medical insurance and permanent health insurance would cost poorer people comparatively more of their incomes.[33]

Box 6.2: Costs

The lessons of America have been learned in Britain. In 1989, while arguments were being had in the NHS, BUPA was busy emulating the HMOs. A strategy document dating from 1989 makes it clear that managing care properly was considered highly important. The document states:

> BUPA has been committed to cost containment, the stabilisation of the rate of growth in premiums both limiting risk coverage. Managed care may be a vital tool in achieving this strategy ... In 1987 BUPA paid 81% of its earned subscriptions in benefit payment. If the managed care proposals were implemented, potential saving in excess of £49 million could be achieved (based on savings of 15%).

A year later a clearer strategy was taking shape after management consultants identified six key areas for achieving savings, of which BUPA concentrated on three-day care, lengths of stay and diagnostic testing procedures.

The report notes: 'significant savings could be achieved by ensuring that whenever appropriate procedures are carried out on a day case basis thus reducing the need for costly overnight accommodation and other associated charges.' The savings are estimated at between £17 and £68 million. It continues. 'There are considerable variations between providers that reflect both pre-operative and continued stay patterns. Considerable savings can be made by ensuring optimum lengths of stay. These are calculated at between £11.5 million and £46.5 million'. It added 'The evidence ... suggests that patients are routinely admitted for diagnostic tests which could be undertaken as an outpatient or in appropriate circumstances as a day case'. The savings here vary from £1.3 million to £5.6 million. In total the savings were estimated to be between £30 million and £120 million. The plan was put into effect, setting up a structure of data collection and reporting. The reporting criteria moved the debate on into a very sensitive area – clinical quality: 'In future reporting on providers will not purely be on a cost profile basis but will also include utilisation reports and quality profiles.'

It also made clear that:

The key to achieving savings through utilisation review is the recognition that although there are wide ranges of clinical practice a reasonable level of concensus can be reached on what constitutes acceptable standards. The process of reviewing ... information and of comparing it both with other clinicians and with recognised authorities on utilisation issues can lead to the development of standards which BUPA can apply when assessing utilisation pattern.

In other words, BUPA was planning to do something that had never officially been done within the NHS – gather information of its own in order to make decisions on how to treat people according to the quality of the doctors and hospitals being used. The measures sound remarkably similar to those on which NHS managers have more recently concentrated to bring their costs under control. However, the effectiveness of these measures is questionable as high costs are still a major problem for the private sector.[34]

Labour

Labour has not addressed the question of whether the NHS is under-funded or not perhaps because the wrong answer – that it is – would lead to a need to make spending commitments where increased spending has been ruled out. The spending environment for health over the next three years is the harshest ever encountered – averaging at an increase of 0.5% a year, where the average rise for the past 15 years has been 3%. Talk of a crisis over the period has been increasing, and there has been £300 million extra allocated to the NHS for 1997–98 to help with winter pressures and £1.2 billion extra pumped into the system for 1998–99 to stave off repeats of 1987. Figures are keeping wolves from doors.[35]

Ruling out specific spending commitments, however, has not meant the Government is not addressing key funding questions. Three interesting policy developments have emerged since it came to power.

The first is that, bowing to Treasury pressure for a comprehensive spending review, Frank Dobson has refused to rule out charging for some NHS services – notably visits to the doctor.[36] The initiative was seized by the BMA who in October 1996 published a paper examining charging, which up until then had been a taboo subject. The growing feeling is that while such moves could be seen as undermining the spirit of the service, it could equally be argued that charges have accompanied some services from their earliest days and that charges need to be broadened and not deepened, as traditionally had been the case. Second, the fact is that it may be better to have a withdrawing from principle in favour of a pragmatic answer to the question: 'Can the NHS survive in any form and if so, which form?' Dobson has also considered a hypothecated health tax but the signs are this will be defeated by the Treasury. That is a shame.

The Government has also promised: 'If you are ill or injured there will be an NHS there to help ... access to it will be based on need and need alone, not on your ability to pay or who your GP happens to be or where you live. Every aspect of our spending review will be judged against these criteria. The criteria will be: would a particular proposal mean that access remained based on need alone or would it mean that access became related to ability to pay? Would the introduction or the increase of a charge put people off seeking the treatment or care that they need?' Clearly there is room for manoeuvre here. Alongside this the DoH was considering extending prescription charges and the Government plans to introduce cash limits for GP drugs budgets. Another development was the report that the Department of Health is considering pressing for a hypothecated health tax.[36]

The third strand of policy is the private finance initiative (PFI). Labour is committed to the PFI, enacting legislation drafted by the last government to enable deals held up by legal problems to be passed, but has made clear it will not allow PFI to cover clinical services.

The Party still seems clear on the question of incentives for private insurance – abolishing the tax break for over 60s taking out PMI. And it has postponed the application of partnership scheme to long-term care, appointing a Royal Commission to investigate the issue.

Aside from these announcements there have been a series of acknowledgements that the NHS faces a funding crisis of the previous Government's making effecting waiting lists and nurses' pay, but that sufficient funds will be made available to cover it providing everyone works together to stem the problems.[36]

In the longer term there are greater problems. As an Institute for Fiscal Studies analysis points out, the concensus before the election on total public spending has serous implications for health care. Ignoring complications caused by transferral of some community care functions from the NHS to local government, the IFS calculates an expected 1.8% increase in funding in 1997/98, zero increase in 1998/99 and 1999/2000 – an average increase of 0.6%.[37]

Of the original spending plans, the IFS says:

Either they are infeasible, and will be broken, or they will mean a much lower injection of new resources into the health service than hitherto experienced. At a time when the public's demand for health care is inevitably rising, this will have serious implications for how well the NHS will be able to continue in its role as a comprehensive universal provider of free health care.

In the event they were broken. Gordon Brown's £1.5 million gift may help at the margins but the fact that the election was won on such spending commitments does not bode well for the future if nothing is changed. The IFS's view should give everyone pause for thought.

References

1 Bevan A (1952) *In Place of Fear*. Heinemann, London.
2 Foot M (1973) *Aneurin Bevan: a biography (Volume 2)*. Davis-Poynter, London.
3 Guillebaud C (1956) *Report of the Committee of Enquiry into the National Health Service* (Cmnd 9663). HMSO, London.
4 Appleby J (1992) *Financing Healthcare in the 1990s*. Open University Press, Buckingham.
5 Klein R (1995) *The New Politics of the National Health Service*. (3rd ed.) Longman, London.
6 Institute of Health Services Management (1997) *Survey of Health Services Managers*. IHSM, London.
7 DoH (1997) *Provisional waiting list figures*. 30 June (press release).
8 For accounts of the health review see Lawson N (1992) *The View from Number 11*. Bantam Press, London: Thatcher M (1993) *The Downing Street Years*. HarperCollins, London; and for an excellent historical analysis Timmins N (1995) *The Five Giants: a biography of the welfare state*. HarperCollins, London.
9 Secretaries of State for Health, Wales, Northern Ireland and Scotland (1989) *Working for Patients* (Cmnd 555). HMSO, London.
10 Harrison S (1995) *The Dynamics of Healthcare Policy*. Institute for Public Policy Research, London.
11 Jowell R, Curtice J, Park A *et al.* (1996) *British Social Attitudes: the 13th report*. Dartmouth Publishing, Aldershot.
12 Mattison N (ed.) (1995) *Sharing the Costs of Health: a multi-country perspective*. Pharmaceutical Partners for Better Healthcare, Basel.
13 Hibbs J and Hall C (1997) Outcry over threat of NHS charges. *Daily Telegraph*. 14 June; Timmins N and Parker G (1997) Labour slated for mooting NHS charges. *Financial Times*. 14 June; DoH (1997) *NHS care available to all, according to need and free at the point of use*. 30 June (press release).
14 Timmins N (1997) NHS charges to be debated by doctors. *Financial Times*. 12 June. Social Market Foundation (1997) *Ready for Treatment*. SMF, London.
15 Timmins N (1997) Spending review may lead to NHS tax. *Financial Times*. 9 June.

16 Mulgan G and Murray R (1993) *Reconnecting Taxation.* Demos, London; Davies S and Chandler D (1994) *Hypothecated Taxation and the Future of Healthcare.* Independent Healthcare Association, London. For a good overview of the debate, see Jones A and Duncan A (1995) *Hypothecated Health Taxes: an evaluation of recent proposals.* Office of Health Economics, London; British Medical Association (1994) *Note on Hypothecated Taxation.* BMA, London.

17 Green D (1996) *Community Without Politics: A market approach to welfare reform.* Institute of Economic Affairs, London; Green D (1995) A Note of Dissent, in *Healthcare 2000: UK Health and Healthcare Services. Challenges and Policy Options.* Healthcare 2000, London.

18 Laing W (1996) *Laing's Review of Private Healthcare, 1996/97.* Laing & Buisson, London.

19 Besley T, Hall J and Preston I (1996) *Private Health Insurance and the State of the NHS.* Institute for Fiscal Studies, London.

20 Green D (1988) *Everyone a Private Patient.* Institute of Economic Affairs, London.

21 Towse A (1995) An overview of the NERA study and its proposals for health-care reform, in A Towse (ed.) *Financing Healthcare in the UK: a discussion of NERA's prototype model to replace the NHS.* Office of Health Economics, London.

22 Laing W (1995) The case for the NERA proposals for reform of the NHS, in A Towse (ed.) *Financing Healthcare in the UK: a discussion of NERA's prototype model to replace the NHS.* Office of Health Economics, London.

23 Culyer AJ (1995) Chisels or Screwdrivers? a critique of the NERA proposals for the reform of the NHS, in A Towse (ed.) *Financing Healthcare in the UK: a discussion of NERA's prototype model to replace the NHS.* Office of Health Economics, London.

24 Interview with David Green, November 1995.

25 Bosanquet N (1995) *Public Spending into the Millennium.* Social Market Foundation, London.

26 Laing & Buisson (1996) *Care of Elderly People: market survey 1996.* (9th ed.) Laing & Buisson, London.

27 Chancellor of the Exchequer, Secretary of State for Social Security, President of the Board of Trade *et al.* (1996) *A New Partnership for Care in Old Age.* HMSO, London.

28 Interview with Age Concern, May 1996.

29 Interview with William Laing, May 1996; see also Laing W (1993) *Financing Long-term Care.* Age Concern, London.

30 Richards E (1996) *Paying for Long-term Care.* Institute for Public Policy Research, London.

31 Macdonald V and Slade P (1996) When insurers say no. *Sunday Telegraph,* 15 September.

32 Office of Fair Trading (1996) *Health Insurance.* Office of Fair Trading, London.

33 Hills J and Burchardt T (1997) *Private Welfare Insurance and Social Security: pushing the boundaries.* Joseph Rowntree Foundation, London.

34 BUPA (1989/90) *BUPA Provider Affairs Centre Briefings.* BUPA, London.

35 HM Treasury (1997) *Financial Statement and Budget Report.* HMSO, London.

36 Timmins N (1997) Dobson admits NHS is facing financial crisis. Financial Times. 9 June; DoH (1997) *Dobson welcomes extra £1 billion for NHS in England.* 2 July (press release); DoH (1997) *Frank Dobson is determined to minimise winter pressures on the NHS.* 12 June (press release).

37 Institute for Fiscal Studies (1997) *Election Briefing.* IFS, London.

7 Hospitals

Hospitals are the castles of the twentieth century. The science of medicine may lag some way behind those of fortification and warfare but hospitals show some of the most important features of medieval military fortification: they are strategically positioned, conspicuous and they are easy to defend.

They can prolong in those who are involved in their planning and use, and those who depend on them for protection, a belief that they are the only barrier against the enemies they were designed to conquer. In the hospital's case, of course, this is disease. The presence of a hospital in every part of the kingdom – thanks to the 1962 hospital plan – presents a united front against the evils of disease and sickness.

A doctor's hospital is his castle, and he will go to great lengths to ensure that it remains standing and expanding. In the face of closure he will generally be supported by his local MP. He will find the public is an easy audience to win over – 'shroud waving' on a public platform with the threat of a closed accident and emergency department looming in the background is a potent device. General practitioner unease will also be easy to exploit, and a garrison of nurses, their employment threatened, will man the battlements and fight for survival.

Battles over district general hospitals threatened with closure are a one-sided affair. Doctors, nurses and their champions, MPs, are seen as heroic fighters against adversity, standing up for the traditional values of the NHS against the ubiquitous cost cutting of efficiency-crazed management. It is an easily stereotyped situation because it is so familiar. From newspaper campaigns to save famous teaching hospitals like St Bartholomew's from closure to local demonstrations to save accident and emergency units, emotion is always loaded fairly and squarely with the campaigners.

The example of Edgware General Hospital, in north London is an interesting case in point. Arguments between managers and doctors over the hospital's accident and emergency unit rumbled on for years, but the hospital made the headlines when two local Conservative MPs threatened to withdraw their support for the then Government if the hospital's future was not guaranteed. With the Conservative majority wafer thin, the action was portrayed as 'holding the Government to ransom'.

The *Daily Telegraph* summed up the situation well, writing:

There will be rejoicing among those who have strenuously campaigned for many months to save the Edgware General Hospital ... Details remain to be settled but it seems clear that thanks to the intervention of two local members of parliament, the Health Secretary, Stephen Dorrell, has made a U-turn and will now grant a reprieve to the hospital's casualty service.[1]

Such is the power of the hospital over the most powerful in the land.

But, according to many analyses, the problem is that the pressures to close hospitals are only ever going to get greater. The city of Derby, for example, hit the headlines when its children's hospital was threatened because of changes in the national funding formula to health authorities. This meant a cut in resources to the city and the need to shuffle services around. Other priorities were seen as greater, so the unit – the first children's hospital to be built in Britain for 90 years – faced the ignominy of the threat of closure before it had even opened.[2]

The health system of the future may rely less and less on the district general hospital. As we saw with our look ahead into the system of 2048, the future could see an array of facilities from the giant super hospital through to health centres and patient hotels. The forces for this kind of system are great.

The question now is whether the network of hospitals handed down from the hospital plan has, like the Maginot line, bred a false sense of security in us. Are hospitals really the proper way of waging war on the modern health battlefield? Or have the forces massed against them changed, so as to render them more harmful and less helpful than in the past?

Pressures for change

The market

The importance of these questions is greater now than ever before. First, despite the fact that it has been limited, the internal market has made the world of health care a more precarious place. Purchasers are unwilling to waste money on services whose costs are inflated because hospital wards are half empty and doctors underutilized. They want mergers to make services more streamlined. While hospital closures are not on the agenda at present, reconfiguration within certainly is. Hospital managers have to be more aware than ever of the need to position themselves correctly in the health marketplace. They need to bring outdated supply networks into line with changing patterns of demand. Even though the market may not be permitted to deliver the rationalizations demanded by efficiency, particularly where hospitals have more than 600 beds and the case for mergers is questioned, there is plenty of management time spent defending individual hospital positions in the marketplace, particularly in the case of individual departments.

Another element of the reforms, allied to the introduction of the market, is the move towards a primary care-led NHS. Primary and community care is seen as cheaper, more sensitive to the consumer and, in political terms, easier to manage than the hospital sector of the NHS.

Demography and technology

Second, there is a series of deep seated changes that is altering what can and should be done inside and outside hospitals. The very nature of the hospital is being questioned. What, after all, is a hospital? A machine for curing people? A place of isolation? A place to monitor long-term illness? A 'workshop' to replace bodily parts? What, moreover is the safest, most efficient and fair way of providing these things? Is it actually in one place, or would the services in a hospital be best split into the community? Would they be cheaper? Would they be safer? Would they be more consumer friendly?

What is clear is that changes in demography and technology have greatly affected demand and supply of health care. Disease patterns have changed, from the infectious diseases of the nineteenth and early twentieth century to the chronic conditions of today – for example, heart disease – and of the future: asthma, AIDS, lung cancer.

As people grow older, so their care needs will differ. As family patterns change, so the contribution of the traditional and free 'informal carer' will decline. Expectations will continue to rise, demanding higher quality. Education will have its impact and, as the population becomes better informed, perceptions of what good health is will alter too.

There will be pressure for services to change. Greater technology will create greater flexibility – miniaturization, information, communication and genetics – as we saw in Chapter 1 – will all have their roles to play. The way services are arranged around demarcations between primary and secondary sectors is likely to shift too.

Technology is revolutionizing health care, and our use of hospitals. Keyhole surgery is leading to a far higher rate of day-case surgery with a corresponding fall in the number of days spent in hospital. The amount of work done on a day surgery basis rose by 150% in the 1980s. Many analysts are now predicting that the jobs and services provided in a hospital will be split up, and certain procedures and services will be moved out into the community, into superstore surgeries or into patient hotels – places for people to wait for operations or convalesce after them, away from the overheads of the 24-hour unit.

These are not new forces. The length of stay in hospitals has declined over many years. For acute care the average has gone down from 6.2 days in 1988 to 4.8 in 1994. For inpatient care as a whole, the figures are more dramatic, falling from 15.6 days in 1990 to 10.2 days in 1993. Beds are working harder. In 1969 each hospital bed in Britain saw some 19.7 acute cases per year. In 1993–94 the figure was 55.4. The outcome: fewer hospital beds are needed. There were 200 000 geriatric and acute beds in 1981; there are 147 000 in 1997.[3]

One study predicts referrals from GPs up the chain to more specialist sites will be reduced by 20%; 40% of outpatient consultations will take place outside the district general hospital; 80% of surgery will be keyhole; 60% of surgery will be day case and acute beds in district general hospitals will be reduced by 40%.[4]

Scenarios like this are very attractive. The idea of receiving top quality care on the high street or in your own home, of leaving the hospital or day care unit within days or on the same day as an operation, the fact that that operation will not have involved opening you up as it would have done 20 years ago, all embody goals that have won widespread support among Ministers and managers.

Financial pressure

Demand on hospital services is growing fast, but these are often inflexible institutions that may not be best suited to dealing with the problems of modern health and social care. In one study some 15 forces on hospitals are identified. They include demographic pressures – with the increasing number of elderly people. Resource pressures, which are feeding through from purchasers who are beginning to demand more reconfiguration. The demand for services is rising continuously, linked to increased public expectations of what the NHS can offer. There are changes in local financial situations, with many health authorities forecasting a reduction in their budgets in the years up to the end of the 1990s because of NHS Executive plans to equalize funding. There are pressures to upgrade capital works in hospital trusts. Coupled with the Government-imposed 3% efficiency targets, this will create pressure for change.[5]

There are many other pressures. The attempts to reduce junior doctors' hours will cut the capacity of services, increasing the pressure to merge services between trusts. The drive for clinical effectiveness also points in the direction of combining some smaller specialties.

Another major factor was the increase in accident and emergency admissions, which has accelerated rapidly in the 1990s, growing by some 13% per annum between 1989 and 1994. At the same time there has been a reduction in the total number of acute beds by some 10% (13 000 beds). The strain is showing in many hospitals.[6]

The implications are widespread. Hospitals have to act faster. The creation of special high-dependency or admissions wards has been suggested as a way of dealing with the problems. This has knock-on effects, with patients shuffled between beds to make room for emergency admissions. Hospitals can actually be temporarily 'closed' to medical admissions – one study found 32% of hospitals had had to take this course, and there are increasing 'trolley waits' as patients queue up for beds.[7]

Equity

The distribution of hospitals, which originated with the hospital plan, has implications for inequity.[8] One level higher in the decision making structure – the hospital management – there are different problems. Although there is coverage by hospitals around the country, the level and quality of and access to services vary greatly. There are major differences in the level of intensive care services around the country, for example, and heart surgery was also found to be variable across the country.[9]

Box 7.1: Hospital drama

Changes to hospitals often create massive conflict for very little result. One particularly tough fight over changing hospital services was in Sheffield. The A&E department in one of the city's two hospitals – the Northern General or the Hallamshire – would have to close. A&E closures are always controversial, not only from the public's point of view who see fewer sites as exposing them to greater risk, but also from clinical staff who see casualty as 'the heart of a hospital'.

Neil Mackay, former Chief Executive of the Trent Region of the NHS Executive, was Chief Executive of the Northern General. His account of the battle between the two hospitals gives a clear indication of the emnity that can exist between institutions when old rivalries are intensified with pressures to rationalize.

Mackay says: 'The Northern General was created out of two hospitals in 1970. It was a teaching hospital, but was always seen as the poor relation in Sheffield, the second rate hospital. The Hallamshire was the number one and had been a teaching hospital from time immemorial.'

Mackay arrived at the Northern General in 1988. He says there had been quite some resentment building up at the hospital about its status relative to the Hallamshire, and relationships with the health authority in Sheffield were not good. 'There was a feeling that the Hallamshire got everything – expensive equipment, any consultant posts, power and influence. The reforms gave us the opportunity we had all been waiting for, a chance to throw off the health authority's influence. We became a trust in the first wave and stole a march on the Hallamshire. We were probably pretty horrible to start with and pretty robust with the way we used our freedoms.'

To begin with there was an argument about urology services in Sheffield. It was decided it would be concentrated on one site – the Hallamshire. Mackay and his staff were bitterly disappointed. 'Then, around about the time that we became a trust the regional health authority decided that A&E services would have to be changed because they cost more in Sheffield than they did anywhere else in the country. We decided we had to change our tactics – over urology we had been horrible to the health authority. When the A&E review came along we were reasonable and the purchaser/provider relationship changed dramatically. We became very amenable, to try and outmanoeuvre the Hallamshire and get in with the health authority. In the end, in 1995, we won the argument – largely, I think, due to this policy. There was a great deal of ill feeling between us and the Hallamshire – after all, the old institution had lost out, and its A&E department had to close. That is important for any hospital.'

The struggle had other implications, too: 'The situation brought the doctors and managers together; they had a common purpose. We had weekly meetings with the senior clinicians throughout the whole process. When we won, I think it reaffirmed our status within the hospital. We had been seen to do our job well. The publicity was awful. There was a lot of leaking and the papers took us to task. At one point the papers printed a front page headline just saying "SHAMBLES". The whole process was portrayed as a muddle with disastrous consequences for Sheffield. The Chief Executive of the other trust had gone to the paper saying that without A&E the Hallamshire would be finished as a hospital, and that would have dire consequences for the city. Of course, that did not turn out to be true.'

Interview with Neil Mackay, September 1996.

Obstacles

But are such changes practical? Are they even desirable? Is the public fear of 'things going wrong' outside hospital justified? In many of the scenarios above the implications for costs are unclear. Breaking up the hospital or replacing the network of district general hospitals with smaller and larger units may have unforeseen consequences. The dynamics of how a hospital operates are anything but clear.

The Hospital Plan

The modern system of hospitals was established after Enoch Powell's 1962 Hospital Plan. Along with it, the modern attitude to the health service was entrenched. As the medieval network of parish churches up and down the country proved the existence of God, the hospitals prove the existence of health care.

The plan was drafted in response to the recognition that the patchwork of voluntary and public hospitals built up since the nineteenth century was not spreading specialist care equally around the country. It was thought that concentration of services in one institution like a district general hospital would be efficient and would provide quality.[8]

It was a serious attempt to break the inequities in the health system. In the words of one civil servant working for Powell at the time:

> There was a feeling that this was the beginning of the real National Health Service. For those in the department there was a feeling that Powell was a great minister of health because he was the first one to get the National Health Service put to the top of the spending pile. Up until then the priorities had been housing and education. I think Bevan would have approved of what the hospital plan achieved.[10]

But there were contradictions running through the plan, and the thinking behind it. The plan was indeed directly in the spirit of the Bevanite NHS – using science and rational planning to spread a fair and equal service across the country. Ninety new hospitals were to be built, 134 upgraded and a total of £500 million was to be spent on them over the next ten years – three times more than the £157 million that had been spent since the service was founded in 1948. Calculations about the size of the hospitals, and the array of local services in which they would stand at the centre were carried out to make it clear that this would provide a system that was not only equitable, but efficient too. Moreover, in launching the hospital plan a political establishment that was only too aware of the power of the medical establishment – and wary of it – had built for that group its own power base. Powell recognized that the hospital doctor was 'king in his castle'.[11]

In fact the plan did not go quite as anticipated. As Klein has noted, NHS building programmes were low in the priorities of vote-maximizing politicians, and ministers of health were happier to see the capital programme cut when the Treasury made demands for savings than seeing the budget for treatment pruned, and doctors themselves preferred spending to fund pay rises.

The Hospital Plan also faced difficulties in its attempt to tackle the quest for equity in the NHS. The provision of district general hospitals across the country had to fit local circumstances if it was to provide a truly equitable service, but there was no information on how communities differed or would differ in future.

The plan's strategy was for every population centre of 100 000 to 150 000 people to have its own 600-to-800-bed district general hospital, in which all but a few highly specialized treatments would be provided. These district general hospitals would represent the middle of a three tiered system, with smaller hospitals providing limited services for the community, like maternity care, and the higher level providing specialized services like cancer. In 1969 the Bonham Carter Report suggested doubling the catchment area for district general hospitals.[12]

The legacy of the plan has been less than universal. The changing nature of the hospital and economic problems have given it a more 'stop-start' character than the smooth, rolling ten-year plans envisaged in 1962. The district general hospital is ubiquitous although the services offered vary considerably around the country.

Small hospitals have, since the 1960s been the poor relations to the service. In 1959 there were 912 hospitals with under 50 beds; there were 421 in 1989–90. Similarly, very large hospitals, with over 1000 beds have fallen from nine to three. Those in the medium range, 510 to 1000 beds have gone up from 76 in 1959 to 105 in 1989–90.[9]

Harrison and Prentice write:

> Even though the 1962 Plan may well be regarded as an appropriate response to the conditions prevailing at the time, in the years since the plan was formulated, the way hospitals function has been radically transformed. None of the specific assumptions made at that time, such as the number of beds needed to service a particular population, remain valid as the technology of hospital care has transformed the way that hospital resources are used.[9]

Some community-based hospitals are now claiming their safety record is better than larger hospitals, which are finding their manpower and workload to be so poorly matched that they are losing their reputation for quality. In one example Queen Mary's, Roehampton, a famous London teaching hospital, lost its teaching status in some specialties because quality was being jeopardized by high workloads.

This is very different from the early days of the hospital plan, where DGHs were seen as the best way of combating unsafe cottage hospitals. Technology may be marching to the rescue, providing flexible local services, but it is also determining that some services must be provided in highly specialist sites.

Welcome to hospital

The front door of a hospital is its accident and emergency department. It will need a number of specialist services – identified in one study as general medicine and surgery, paediatrics, trauma and orthopaedics, obstetrics and gynaecology, radiology, anaesthetics, intensive care and coronary care – to back up this central service.

But hospitals offer a much wider variety of services than this list. The interrelation between all specialties and subspecialties in hospitals is complex, and complications in planned operations mean that concentration on one site of all these capabilities has been seen as vital.

Economies of scale?

Economies of scale exist in sharing expensive items of equipment across specialties and avoiding having to duplicate them across more than one hospital. One site may also reduce NHS and patient transport costs and management costs.

American studies have shown how the costs of treating patients fall over time. In one the costs of heart transplants were measured over four years. The fiftieth case was less than one third the cost of the first.[13] In another, neurosurgeons who did a lot of work kept their patients in hospital for fewer days than low volume ones, at a saving of $2000. And in this country, experienced staff were found to take less theatre time. Costs could be reduced by 11.3% if the most experienced staff carried out all operations.

However, internal relationships become more complex and more difficult to manage the larger and more diverse the hospital becomes. And the costs of travelling to the hospital may rise – both to the patient and the NHS in ambulance costs and so on, and in terms of care. The time it takes to get to hospital can crucially affect the survival chances of accident victims.

Neither is the exact nature of economies of scale apparent. Harrison and Prentice point out that as the size of a hospital increases so do the number of wards, and thus, so does the use of its most costly element – nursing.

Co-ordination

It is also unclear which services can be split off from the hospital and better provided in the community. Simpler, low-risk services, like diagnosis, radiology and pathology, and some parts of maternity, elective surgery, even some elements of accident and emergency – in nurse staffed treatment centres like in Westminster – may qualify. The hospital may do things that are already being done in the community – many say that up to 40% of accident and emergency treatments could be carried out in GP surgeries and health centres closer to home and complain that A&E is increasingly used inappropriately. But there are complications around transferring services to the community. Co-ordination between the hospital and GP, and between health authority and local authority social services departments has often been very poor. Further fragmentation could increase the problem.

These tensions already show themselves in problems such as blocked beds. This occurs when patients in an acute bed in a hospital cannot be moved on into the community because social services or nursing home beds cannot be found for them. The reasons for the problems are many, ranging from lack of plans for discharging patients, to lack of co-ordination with social services, to inappropriate admission to hospital in the first place.

In 1996 this was a problem for Fazakerley hospital, which faced difficulties in admitting new patients because its beds were full of elderly people who were ready for discharge into local authority community care but for whom there were no community beds. Sefton, the local authority, claimed it did not have the budget to meet the demand for beds – which cost only £400 a week compared with £1200 in the NHS – and had to push waiting lists back into the hospital. Part of the problem lies in the separate budgets and separate administrations of local authority and NHS beds, which is compounded by the pressure put on the system by the increasing number of people wanting to use it.[14]

In the past, the service was more co-ordinated, with the institutions into which patients were discharged easily accessible from hospital, but the fragmentation of the service through the reforms has broken many of the links, and the discharge procedures needed to link the increasingly disparate elements of the service are in many cases lacking. These systems need to be put in place before the acute, community and primary sector can move into line with each other.[15]

Safety and quality

The district general hospital is such a complex institution that research is ambiguous about whether there would be any danger in taking it apart. As a Department of Health report into cancer services indicated, specialist functions may best be dealt with through facilities that reflect the prevalence of particular conditions. In the case of cancer this would mean having units in district general hospitals that dealt with commoner forms of the disease. For less common forms there would be specialized units, covering larger sections of the population, deriving enough work to ensure doctors kept well practised and up to date and ensuring high quality treatment. In such a hierarchical structure there is a compromise between geographical access, economy and quality. Similar arguments have been made for other services, for example cardiology, although some, like neurosurgery, have too few consultant posts to be provided anywhere outside highly specialist sites.

Anecdotal evidence from GPs suggests there are serious problems within hospitals. The rates of deaths in small hospitals compared with large vary across specialties. So, in an American study, for open heart surgery 38% more people died than would have done if they had been treated in a large hospital, whereas the figure for surgery to sever the vagus nerve to prevent it producing acid in the stomach is only 17%.[16] Whether the cause of a high-quality care is the individual doctor or the hospital is difficult to disentangle.

One study questioned the acceptability and safety of day surgery, minimal access surgery and hospital-at-home schemes to patients. It pointed to problems such as the varying standards of housing that patients were discharged to – a high standard was necessary if day care was to be acceptable. Variable housing meant variable experiences of recuperation – and an indirect effect on the equity of the system. The study found that some patients thought they made a better and faster recovery at home, that they did not think inpatient care was necessary, and that by having day surgery they could free up beds for those who needed them more.

On the other hand, some felt they were going home too soon, without fully recovering from anaesthetic, were anxious about things going wrong at home, that they might not get enough rest there, or that they were being too demanding on relatives. Similar reservations were expressed over hospital-at-home schemes, where patients were keen to convalesce at home if it was possible and comfortable, but would otherwise prefer to remain in the security and comfort of hospitals.[17]

Public opinion

Lastly, the public is attached to its local hospital. People may not see why there are arguments for its closure or for closing some departments. Their confidence in the service may be determined by the bricks and mortar from which their hospital is made. The hospital is the physical evidence that the health system is there for all.

Reconfiguration in practice

The best known of the wide-ranging service reviews was the 1992 Tomlinson Report into hospital services in London.[18] The report argued that more resources needed to be put into primary and community services in London to bring standards up to other parts of the country. Alongside this it found there was likely to be 'a significant fall in the requirement for inpatient beds in inner London hospitals'. This was for two reasons: decline in referrals from outside London as patients were treated more locally, and the increasing efficiency with which beds were being used. Two thousand to 7000 beds would be surplus by the end of the decade. The report reflected how the clustering of old and distinguished institutions was not appropriate to modern health needs. But it trampled on many toes.

The report recommended changes that would reduce the number of beds, focusing on hospitals that were already in trouble due to lack of demand for their services. Special hospital services would have to be reformed. The report led to controversial recommendations threatening some of the oldest hospitals in the country. Tomlinson's recommendations have not been fully implemented, however, due to the public outcry that followed them and the resistance of local MPs to closures caused by decisions made in Westminster and Whitehall. The report also lost credibility when the report's Chairman Sir Bernard Tomlinson himself suggested he may not have had all the evidence he needed.[19]

Tomlinson recommended the merging of University College Hospital and the Middlesex Hospital on the UCH site, merging St Bartholomew's and the Royal London on the Royal London site, merging St Thomas's and Guys on one site and a rationalization in West London.

Similar developments are occurring around the country as purchasers look into the future and see possible shortfalls in funding caused by the organization of their hospitals. In Bristol a review conducted from 1994 onwards looked at accident and emergency, acute services, day case treatment, outpatient treatment, primary care and health promotion services, arguing they needed to be shuffled between several existing sites to be used most efficiently. The health authority responsible – Avon Health – believed it would face a funding gap of some £30 million within ten years unless duplications were avoided and savings made. Its answer was to move services out of acute care.[20]

The reforms have focused similar pressures all around the country. In Newcastle, for example, an acute services review was carried out, but both the city's major hospitals would remain providers. New kinds of service provision were introduced, with Newcastle General Infirmary bringing GPs in to work alongside consultants – breaking down the traditional staff barriers. A new mental health trust was formed, and savings of some £10 million a year for the review would be ploughed into primary care. In Lincoln the amount of money coming through capitation formulae is likely to reduce. Reviews have taken place in more than 20 further areas around the country.[7]

According to a senior member of the NHS Confederation, reconfiguration can only grow in the NHS.

The hospital down the road where the ambulance goes may become a thing of the past for many people. There will be increasing reconfiguration as resources are stretched by the current pattern of things. Many trusts are going to find it difficult remaining viable without being incorporated or merged with or swallowing parts of others. There may be massive savings to be made in the conurbations. One of the results of this will be growing monopoly – where there is efficiency you are likely to find greater monopoly.[21]

But the forces for reconfiguration are often obstructed by local and national interests. The Government responded to Tomlinson in 1993 by accepting the proposals but calling for more research. The methodology of the report was criticized, but the Government pressed ahead with several of the recommendations, announcing in 1995 the merging of St Bartholomew's Hospital, development of St Thomas's hospital as a major specialist centre, with its twin Guys concentrating on local services, and the running down of Edgware Hospital. These recommendations are still pending – and, in the case of Edgware, the Conservative Government backtracked.

On the other hand, Government can prevent reconfiguration – as it did by telling Camden and Islington Health Authority not to move contracts away from University College Hospital in London so as not to disturb reconfiguration. It is another example of how the market is inhibited. As Chris Ham says:

> By intervening to determine the future of health care in London, Ministers were acknowledging the realities of a national health service in which ultimate responsibility for decisions rested with politicians in Westminster. Yet in so doing they ran the risk of weakening the competitive incentives designed to drive down costs and raise standards.[22]

As the opening sections of this chapter have shown, there is also evidence that in practice the picture is far more complicated than theoretical analysis suggests. According to the NHS Centre for Reviews and Dissemination increased volume has been overestimated in terms of its impact on quality of care or outcomes, and there is no evidence to suggest that cost savings come from increasing the number of hospitals with 200 plus beds or that concentrating services reduces access for patients.[23]

Box 7.2: Hospitals

The practical problems indicating the lack of power purchasers have over providers are graphically illustrated in the attempts to reconfigure services in Bristol – and echo the problems hospital managers have in managing change. Jill Turner, Acute Services Planner for Avon Health, recalls them at work throughout the three-year process of reviewing the city's health care services.

'We started the review in 1994, looking ten years into the future and asking what is going to be required.' The factors taken into account in the review included the impact of demographic change, particularly the increase in the number of people over the age of 75. Advancing technology, increasing day surgery, growth of care that could be provided in the community, the needs of teaching and research and the requirement to target health at areas of relative deprivation also contributed. There were financial pressures too. The rising cost of health care and the need to develop and improve services caused concern. Bristol had had ten years of minimal growth in funding, with a further five years of the same in store. The authority was still 3.5% above the capitation target – so the future was gloomy. And trusts were finding it increasingly difficult to cope with cost pressures.

Jill Turner explained that a thorough review of services was undertaken between the major providers in the area, which covers a population of

840 000. The largest was the United Bristol Health Care Trust (UBHT) with £105 million of annual revenue, followed by Southmeads Health Services Trust – £85 million – and Frenchay Health Care Trust – £66 million – both district general hospitals on the outskirts of Bristol. In addition there were the smaller Weston Area Health Care Trust near Weston-Super-Mare – £22 million – and the area's ambulance trust – £7 million.

Turner says:

> We looked at eight acute specialities. We had to fit our services into the financial position we felt we would be facing in the future, but this was not the driving factor behind change. There were a number of other important factors, chiefly that we wanted to increase the quality of care.
>
> We consulted extensively with doctors in all the specialities. In paediatrics we had unanimous advice from all the doctors across Bristol that the services should be brought together in one place instead of being spread out across the city. Again in accident and emergency the clinical advice was unanimous – we did not need three 24 hour A&E departments. We don't have the correct medical backup in some specialities in the smaller hospitals, and patient outcomes would be better if we focused on one site. For instance in Leicester, a city the same size as Bristol, there is only one A&E department.

At the outset of the consultation, the medical staff were all in favour of a change in services. Ironically, in view of what happened, the purchasers were not so sure.

'Actually, we, as purchasers did not want to go ahead with the A&E proposals because we thought they would be too emotive,' says Jill Turner. 'But we were persuaded that for reasons of clinical quality this was the best thing to do.'

The accident and emergency figures were analysed. Frenchay and Southmeads had on average one patient per hour during the night time. Avon Health thought that could be managed at UBHT. This fitted in with paediatrics – which had to be there for accident and emergency, so it seemed the right move. In gynaecology, Frenchay did not have obstetrics, but Southmeads did, so the authority thought it should stay there. In clinical haematology, both Southmeads and UBHT provide inpatient care. This should ideally be provided on one site – again for care quality reasons. Turner thought leukaemia was moving closer to oncology, and there was a big oncology unit at UBHT. So that pointed to moving that service to UBHT.

Turner says her team also saw that rheumatology inpatient work should be brought together. Southmeads had a very big orthopaedics department, which meant rheumatology would make sense there. Cardio-thoracic work needed to go to one site. This has to go with accident and emergency, which pointed to UBHT. Ear nose and throat had to be brought together. A large proportion of that work is done on children, paediatrics were to be at UBHT, so it made sense to move ENT there too. Maxillofacial and oral (plastic surgery and surgery for facial injuries) was to go out to tender.

'Bristol exploded,' says Turner.

> We were completely isolated. There was a media campaign called 'Hands Off Our A&E'. The papers, and people writing into them argued that A&E was needed at Frenchay and Southmeads. Because we had not gone all the way with the doctors – who wanted to move all A&E on to one site, we had alienated them as well.

The doctors were in a difficult position, compromised professionally and by their trust loyalties, says Turner:

> In the beginning they were very good – they took off their trust hats and worked with us to build a more rational pattern of services across the city. But once we had come up with our proposals they backtracked and resumed their loyalties to their trusts. We could not get doctors to come and share platforms with us while we were trying to explain.
>
> Sometimes it was worse. At Southmeads they decided they did not want to lose paediatrics. The clinicians did not support us, and there was a campaign involving all the local primary school headmistresses arguing that paediatrics must remain at Southmeads. Haematology was another emotive area. There was a campaign involving clinicians at Southmeads with very emotive marches through the streets. A lot of these services were safe in terms of jobs, it was just loyalty to their trusts.

Once they could no longer rely on the doctors as allies, the managers found themselves having to make their case alone, without the credibility doctors would have leant them.

'What is very difficult for purchasers in situations like these is getting independent advice', says Turner:

> We're just seen as bureaucrats who want to cut costs. The public poses a problem too. Their attitude is that services in three hospitals are necessarily better than services in one. They could not understand the concepts of services being delivered better in the way we were suggesting. You can't point to improved clinical standards like you can to a hospital extension. It is an act of faith on their part, and one they are often, as we found out, very unwilling to make.

Throughout the process, it was the acute services that people concentrated on. Consideration of other services that were included in the review – mental health, health promotion and primary care and learning difficulties were largely ignored. After the consultation programme, the health authority decided to compromise.

Jill Turner says:

We decided we would give up on accident and emergency and paediatrics, and try to go ahead with everything else. At the time everyone thought Avon Health had come away battered and bruised – and in a sense A&E was a major part of the programme. But interestingly since April 1995 – after the consultation, the doctors have changed again, and come back to us. They have found the combination of a reduction in junior doctors' hours after the recommendations by Kenneth Calman has given them less flexibility – made worse by having three sites – and that his recommendations on training and on cancer services have had similar impacts. If everything is on one site it is easier to arrange junior doctor cover, you don't have to shuffle so many different juniors around so many sites. You can have the right people in the right place at the right time.

The review is still being implemented – slowly.

The implications of the Bristol reorganization were widespread and the relationships between the parties rocky and complex. However, a number of smaller scale reorganizations – for example in Kingston and Richmond, where inpatient treatment has been moved to one site and agreement on sharing expensive equipment, and arrangements across two sites was agreed, and Salford and Trafford where ENT services have been moved around – were undertaken without too many problems.[20]

Labour

The pressures of change, coupled with the impact of reform, itself responding to those pressures, suggests that the current backbone of hospitals must be altered if it is to sustain the system in future.

In order to deal with fragmentation, the government recognizes the need to think about local services in a co-ordinated way with its proposals for health action zones – (HAZs). These would break down 'Berlin Walls' between local agencies – health authorities, trusts, GPs and community nurses and local authorities.

The Government says that in the HAZs (possibly numbering ten) 'All those involved in delivering the NHS on the ground would be brought together to develop a health strategy in co-operation with community groups, the voluntary sector, and local businesses.' This must also involve reconfiguration of departments and services and trial integration with local authority social services departments to complement joint commissioning pilots. Tony Blair has also made clear that much of the £300 million extra for the health service will be spent on paying for extra social service accommodation to ease bed blocking.

The Government also promoted the HAZ scheme as a move towards co-operation, and away from 'crack pot competition'. It added that the broadening of health into other agencies may allow funds to be shifted from other departments.

The Government acknowledges the need for rationalization of trusts and said that HAZs could lead the way to a new phase of hospital mergers, but it added that the views of local people would be sought before changes to hospitals were carried out. Whatever consultation strategy is decided upon is likely to be criticized along the lines set out in Chapter 5.[24]

Interestingly, managers at the 1997 NHS Trust conference showed their support for well-managed hospital closures. One trust chief executive said: 'I am sure there are too many hospitals around the country and they are not sufficiently flexible.'[25] It is unclear whether she included her hospital (in Scunthorpe) among these.

The Government also put the London hospital review on the back burner appointing a new review group under Sir Leslie Turnberg, president of the Royal College of Physicians. The group would review what Tomlinson had reviewed, advising in particular on St Bartholomews, Queen Mary's Roehampton, Harold Wood and Oldchurch hospitals.

It was also charged with reviewing health authority plans for 1998–99, ensuring the Government's priorities were being met. The terms of reference – to ensure quality primary care, continuing care, mental health services, co-ordination and A&E – are very similar to Tomlinson. Presumably, however, a different result is hoped for, which is a strong possibility given the background of the chairman. Tomlinson was a businessman.

Nevertheless, the Government seems determined to appear tough in other areas. Alan Milburn launched a fresh autumn 'drive' to merge NHS trusts in 1997, claiming each one would save the NHS £500 000 and aiming for 16, involving 30 hospitals, by April 1998. He added that mergers, along with strengthened health authorities would be a theme of the White Paper.[26]

However, the blanket use of mergers was criticized in the *Financial Times* by Alan Maynard, the leading health economist, who claimed that not all mergers, particularly those involving larger hospitals, would save money. 'As you get bigger, you do not necessarily save money. You get more problems, your capacity to control what is going on diminishes. Managers are thinned out across different sites and have less ability to manage. Before there is a widespread merger policy, each merging trust had better be very sure it is going to make savings before it goes ahead.'[27]

References

1 Leader (1996) A government in casualty. *Daily Telegraph*. June 14.
2 Ward D (1996) First childrens' hospital may have to close. *Guardian*. Sept 3.
3 OECD (1996) *Health Data*. OECD, Paris.
4 Warner M and Riley C (1994) *Closer to Home: healthcare in the 21st century*. NAHAT, Birmingham.
5 Turner J (1994) *Current Issues in Acute Care I: reconfiguring acute services*. Institute of Health Services Management, London.
6 Moore W (1995) *Emergency Admissions: the management challenge*. NAHAT, Birmingham.
7 Turner J (1995) *Current Issues in Acute Care: reconfiguring acute services II*. Institute of Health Services Management, London; Turner J (1996) *Current Issues in Acute Care: reconfiguring acute services III*. Institute of Health Services Management, London.
8 See Minister of Health (1962) *A Hospital Plan for England and Wales* (Cmnd 1604). HMSO, London.
9 Harrison A and Prentice S (1996) *Acute Futures*. King's Fund, London, p. 7.
10 Interviews, August/September 1996.
11 Powell JE (1975) *Medicine and Politics*. (2nd ed.) Pitman Medical, London.
12 DHSS (1969) *The Functions of the District General Hospital*. HMSO, London.
13 Woods J, Saywell R Jnr, Nyhins A *et al*. (1992) The learning curve and the cost of heart transplants. *Health Services Research*. 1: 27.
14 Interview with Fazakerley Hospital management, 1996.
15 Marks L (1994) *Seamless Care or Patchwork Quilt: discharging patients from acute hospital care*. King's Fund Institute, London.
16 Luft H *et al*. (1990) *Hospital Volume, Physician Volume and Patient Outcomes: assessing the evidence*. Health Administration Press Perspectives, Ann Arbor, MI.
17 Henwood M (1995) *Tipping the Balance*. NAHAT, Birmingham.
18 Tomlinson B (1992) *Report of the Inquiry into London's Health Service, Medical Education and Research*. HMSO, London.
19 Revill J (1995) Tomlinson tells of regrets over Bart's facts he never saw. *Evening Standard*. 8 June.
20 Interview with Jill Turner, Avon Health Authority, September 1996.
21 Interview with Eric Morton, NAHAT, September 1996.
22 Ham C (1997) *Management and Competition in the NHS*. (2nd ed.) Radcliffe Medical Press, Oxford.
23 Centre for Reviews and Dissemination (1997) *Concentration and Choice in the Provision of Hospital Services*. Centre for Reviews and Dissemination, University of York.

24 DoH (1997) 'Health Action Zones' envisaged as co-operative NHS partnerships. 25 June (press release).
25 Quoted in Health Service Journal. July 3, p. 12.
26 Timmins N (1997) Drive to merge NHS trusts launched. Financial Times. 22 September.
27 Interview with Alan Maynard, September 1997; see also NHS Centre for Reviews and Dissemination (1997) Hospital Mergers Report. NHS Centre for Reviews and Dissemination, York.

8 Evidence and effectiveness

The cornerstone of a national health system must be the effectiveness of the treatment it offers. If treatment is ineffective, the system is wasting time, money, effort and is probably dangerous too. Such principles seem so self-evident and straightforward as to be beyond question. And so they remained for decades, even centuries, as health care passed through the various stages of its evolution, passing knowledge acquired through ages of experience. Once they were questioned, however, some difficult problems emerged.

Archie Cochrane

The father of the movement for 'evidence-based medicine' was the celebrated epidemiologist Archie Cochrane. Cochrane, like his colleague Thomas McKeown, was a medical sceptic. He argued that no more money should be spent on health care until research methods improved drastically. Cochrane believed that the NHS was hamstrung by its research, that it was not concentrating on treatments that were effective because it did not know which ones those were, and that it was therefore wasting money. He bases his view on three strands. The first, a nod to McKeown, questioned the claims of medicine that it had defeated disease, recognizing the great role public health had played in the health of the nation. The second was the placebo effect, which made it difficult to isolate whether it was the doctor or the patient who was responsible for the success or failure of treatment.

The most important point, however, was the last. Cochrane believed the culture of research in the NHS was misguided. The problems of research dated to the nineteenth century when, he wrote: 'For reasons that are still somewhat obscure, British science divided itself into pure and applied, and decided that pure research was "U" and applied research "non-U". This division has had a very detrimental effect on large aspects of British life.'

He continued, recalling his day as a medical student at Cambridge:

I remember being advised by the most distinguished people that the best research should be utterly useless. The importance of this to my present arguments is best illustrated by the situation when the NHS was introduced. This was a national organisation which from one point of view could be seen as giving a blank cheque both to the demands of patients and the wishes of doctors. Most industrial organisations of comparable size would have had a large research section checking on the effectiveness of the service it was providing. In point of fact there was no research of this kind for about the first fifteen years of the life of the NHS.[1]

Cochrane is worth quoting at length because his arguments are still informing debate today. There is now a research and development department at the Department of Health. Sir Michael Peckham, its former Director, on leaving his post in January 1996, said at least £1 billion could be saved by cutting out unnecessary and ineffective treatments in the NHS.[2]

The standard of research was important to Cochrane. His goal was to see a 'gold standard' applied across the NHS. The gold standard was the 'randomised controlled trial' in which treatments would be checked against a carefully selected group of people to isolate the purely medical effects from demographic, social and other influences. By dividing the group in two randomly, treatments can be compared with each other.

Cochrane believed that British medicine was miles from such a rational and scientific approach. He said the most common form of evidence was the oldest – clinical opinion – but he said: 'its value must be rated low, because there is no quantitative measurement, no attempt to discover what would have happened if the patients had had no treatment, and every possibility of bias affecting the assessment of the result'. Next up the line were comparison groups which he considered often to be 'grotesque' for their lack of science.

Cochrane argued that the lack of a scientific approach affected not only the quality of treatment but the cost of the system through massive waste and inefficiency. He pointed the finger at the BMA, which was unwilling to change traditional practice to control costs: 'No one I am sure can visualise the BMA with its slogan of "clinical freedom" controlling the doctors.'[1]

Evidence-based medicine (EBM) today

Cochrane's prognosis for the future of the NHS makes fascinating reading today. The measures he espouses are still widely advocated. EBM has found its way into the medical mainstream. Even today's BMA chairman, Dr Sandy Macara, lauds him saying: 'He was 20 years ahead of his time.'[3]

Health economists still follow his views in large part because they do not believe his work is finished. Alan Maynard of the University of York maintains that only 20% of treatments regularly carried out in the NHS are based on rigorously scientific evidence-based tests.[4] Others have unproven effectiveness, not to mention cost effectiveness, and may do more harm than good. He argues that medical training fills students full of facts without asking them to understand the basis on which these facts are founded. Gwyn Bevan and Brendan Devlin, an economist and an eminent surgeon write: 'It is a truism that much of medical care has not been evaluated, so its benefits are not known. When doctors decide to admit an individual to hospital they often do so without firm evidence that this will be more effective than doing nothing.'[5]

The point of EBM is neatly summed up: 'In essence, evidence-based medicine involves a shift in the culture of health care provision, away from basing decisions on opinion, past practice and precedent and towards making more use of science, research and evidence to guide decision making.'[6]

There is a long way to go. Many treatments viewed as ineffective are still widely carried out. The kind of treatment carried out by doctors and hospitals around the country varies, with a lack of standardization. There are clinical guidelines, but their effectiveness and ease of application is open to question. All of these problems militate against attempts to impose scientific order on the system.

If any of the work on evidence-based care is to find its way into practice it must be accepted by the commissioning authorities. Purchasing evidence-based care has developed since the outset of the reforms. A 44 page booklet of guidance notes from the Department of Health points to the need for information to be available, for it to be incorporated into local planning by health authorities and for it to be monitored for feedback. It lists the sources of available evidence and suggests that its register of cost effective studies will be expanded from the small number of treatments it covers to encompass medical practice and show what should and should not be brought by the NHS.[7]

Some doctors are finding their hand is being forced. Purchasers are taking the initiative and refusing to pay for some treatments.

The Government has invested in promoting evidence-based medicine, setting up a research and development department in the NHS, and explicitly requiring health purchasers to include evidence-based criteria in their purchasing patterns in order to identify effective treatments and to stop wasting money on ineffective ones. The previous Government produced documents outlining how authorities can make best use of the material being provided by various centres looking into producing evidence-based guidelines. Progress has, however, been slow with only two evidence-based purchasing decisions required to be made and two ineffective treatments to be taken off the lists.

The results of a lack of a scientific, evidence-based approach mean that health care can become a lottery. This points to another problem – variation in medical practices. In a study by Bevan and Devlin, wide variations between treatments given for the same complaints were found throughout the country.

For example in 1984 admission rates in 135 English health authority districts varied by more than three times for seven common medical conditions from hip replacement to heart attack. Another review in 1990 found that referral rates from GPs around Britain varied by three or fourfold and could not be explained by casemix. Devlin and Bevan also level their sights at grommets for children with glue ear. Despite the use of these treatments being highly questionable, they suggest that ear, nose and throat doctors are looking for ways to keep themselves busy. They say: 'Although the fashion for tonsillectomies as a "cure" for tonsillitis has largely passed, ENT surgeons have replaced this with the "epidemic" of operations for glue ear.'

Bevan and Devlin's study points to the major resource implications of the widespread use of inappropriate treatments. Doctors like to have things to do, and while they have managed to reduce the amount of time people stay in hospital – cutting the duration of expensive hospital stays, and therefore costs – they have increased the volume of services they provide. Many of these are inappropriate. They take Cochrane's line on the implications of all this for health service funding. 'The argument about underfunding of the NHS would be more convincing if we were confident that all NHS care was effective.' They continue: 'What we need to address is not the underfunding of the health service but the underfunding of research and development.'[5]

Barriers to change

The medical tradition

Sir Michael Peckham says that challenging the doctors and their practices is part of the point of EBM:

> I see evidence based medicine as an education for doctors, who need to reappraise what they do, and to question the way they have learned. A

lot of education is based on anecdote. The message seems to me to be that there is a need to shift radically the whole of health care from an empirical basis to a rational one. What we have now is the end product of the history of health care.

And he argues that EBM can be used alongside league tables to measure performance: 'Ideally I would like to see every DGH and tertiary hospital producing some measurable statement of benefits in relation to investments. Then it should be possible to see the differences between them.'[8]

The closer we look into EBM, however, the more obscure its contribution to the NHS's future becomes. First there is major resistance from elements of the medical profession, who see the clinical guidelines and protocols it would introduce as limiting their clinical freedom. Indeed when the subject is raised with doctors, eyes inevitably turn to heaven. One GP said: 'evidence based medicine is cookbook medicine. Medicine should be about the individual, leaving the doctor to work out the correct treatment given the specific conditions of the patient. To take that away would be destroying one of the great strengths of medicine.' Another senior registrar said: 'what do people mean by it? I would have thought most of what I do is evidence based. Anyway, it would turn us all into robots. Doctors are thinking people, they need to research and solve problems themselves.'

While Appleby, Walshe and Ham's definition of EBM seems reasonable enough, others have found it necessary to publish whole articles explaining it. In one, entitled 'Evidence based medicine: what it is and what it isn't', five experts set out the ground. The reason they go to the trouble is interesting. They see EBM as under threat: 'Criticism', they write, 'has ranged from evidence based medicine being old hat to it being a dangerous innovation perpetrated by the arrogant to serve cost cutters and suppress clinical freedom.' It also warns that input from clinicians is important to avoid the 'tyranny' of evidence.[9]

Difficulty in drawing up protocols

But there is another problem with protocols apart from their unpopularity with the medical profession. Even if the objections of doctors can be overcome, the implementation of the evidence has to be done through written guidelines. Studies have shown that the absorption of new evidence by GPs and hospital doctors is too slow to allow EBM to be held up as some form of panacea to all our health ills.[6,10] It is a long-term problem.

Missing the point – clinical audit

Clinical audit involves measuring the activity of doctors in the service. In commercial companies, auditing procedures should be capable of measuring the quality, quantity and cost of the activity of the workforce.

Not so in the NHS. The intentions of clinical audit – to set in place and use yardsticks for monitoring the performance of doctors – can trace their origins back to the eighteenth century, when George II's physician, Francis Clifton, declared that the measurement of hospital performance should be published in an annual report. Audit's modern origins can be traced in the ineffective Cogwheel Reports on management in the NHS. Written between 1967 and 1974, the three reports in the series proposed a management system in which medical specialties came together in divisions to form a medical executive committee to examine hospital services, and to decide how to allocate resources and set priorities in hospitals.[11]

In the same way that job plans had been introduced under the 1990 reforms, so was audit. Hospitals applying for trust status had to have audit procedures in place if they were to succeed, and Royal Colleges were encouraged to include audit as a precondition for hospitals to gain teaching status. The then family health services authorities were to spearhead an audit initiative in primary care.[12]

Theory and practice, however, as so often in the NHS, failed to match up. Rudolf Klein states that audit, 'turned out to be an example of the medical profession's ability to modify – if not to subvert – the government's intentions during the processes of implementation.'[13]

The 'modification' was skilfully and tactically managed by the profession. As a National Audit Office report shows, audit has spread far and wide. It said there were an estimated 20 000 audit initiatives in the NHS in 1993–94, and that 83% of hospital and community health consultants attended most or all clinical audit activities for their specialties, and that most specialties were involved. It also found that 86% of general practices were participating in audit in 1993–94.

The report also stated there were some benefits to patients. Audit was helping doctors to promote clinical guidelines – used to set down best practice for dealing with specific conditions. Audit also helped with identifying good, cost effective practice, improving education, team working and communication, helped provide management with information on quality, and helped provide commissioners with quality information too. Some trusts that had introduced audit also said they had seen increased efficiency after it was implemented.[14]

This is all good. It does not, however, get to the root of the problem. Any manager would like to analyse the outcomes of treatment carried out by hospital doctors – it is part of the trio of measures that management must be able to control: cost, volume and quality. Low cost and high volume are worth nothing if quality is bad, particularly in a service like the NHS. Like any other professional, a doctor who is producing poor results is likely to cost more money in the long run. His work is likely to be inefficient, quite apart from causing distress to or even endangering his patients.

The need for outcomes

Poor medical practice has major ethical implications too. Health care concerns our quality of life, if not always the quantity of it. Outcomes, however, have not been on the audit agenda. Commenting on four reports surveying clinical audit, published by the NHS Executive in 1993 and 1994, the National Audit Office report states: 'the reports concluded clinical audit had led to significant changes in clinical practice and organisation, but they did not set out to assess the impact of clinical audit on the quality of patient care or outcomes.' It went on to say the initiatives were concerned with the delivery of care, not in the outcomes of care.[14,15]

For critics of the medical profession managing the 'delivery' of health care can only have a marginal effect on how efficiently and fairly it can be delivered. By playing the audit game to the limited degree that they are doing, doctors can claim to managers they are co-operating while not doing so at all. As Professor Alan Maynard points out:

Most hospital activity data does not end in death but in changed quality of life. The reluctance of clinicians and managers to measure routinely the impact of health care interventions on the physical, social and psychological functioning of patients is ubiquitous. If hospitals are to demonstrate success how can they continue to be so negligent?[4]

In John Spiers's words: 'All roads lead to outcomes.' For Spiers purchasing must influence medical practice. High-quality, hard information must be available on the effects of treatment. Data must not just record whether someone dies soon after treatment, but must measure the effects of treatment on quality of life over a longer period of time. Flexible clinical protocols must be introduced, so that doctors agree how to treat certain conditions effectively. The purchaser then knows how money is being spent. Doctors must be on board the initiatives – indeed they must spearhead them within hospitals if they are to work. Spiers says: 'Outcomes push us all into managing for performance, managing for improved health status, analysing results patient by patient, procedure by procedure, clinician by clinician, which is how purchasers will soon want to buy.' He points to a possible future where purchaser pressure could lead to 'payment on outcome', so only successful treatments would be reimbursed, and league tables could be constructed on outcome data.[16] This, however, is pushing too far.

In the past, information has been scarce. Suppliers of health care in Britain have not had to worry about demand, or try to measure it. As the NHS is a third-party system funded from general taxation, the person whose pocket was being lightened by any particular decision – the taxpayer – was distant and unable to complain. Now, with purchasers of care responsible for assessing the health needs of their patient lists or resident populations, and responsible for paying to have those needs met, they have a much greater interest in demand and whether or not it is necessary to satisfy it.

Information, then, is at the heart of fundamental change in the influence of purchasers. The key, however, is what kind of information. The above focus – on how much of what is being produced, and how cheaply is a start. But in the minds of many managers, it can only really have a marginal impact on performance if the system it is measuring is not producing effective results. This points to two specific areas – measuring the outcomes of what doctors do and being sure that what they are doing is proven to be effective and safe.

However, despite the greater availability of information Dr Sandy Macara, chairman of the British Medical Association, believes that concentrating on outcomes is missing the point of audit and ignores the great advances made by the medical profession in recent years, threatening those advances by trying to take one step too far. 'In retrospect the medical profession has been desperately slow', Macara says. 'Why did it take 10 years before the BMA started to get involved in audit, and support it?'

He continues:

Of course the BMA wants to be seen to be helping, but there was a great deal of trepidation about accountability. We resisted audit, we resisted any involvement in managing resources, we were suspicious of computer, and of wider availability of, information. The reason was we feared the use to which it would all be put.

But since the battles of the 1970s and 1980s there has been a sea change. The BMA has become involved in pioneering audit. We are involved in the National Centre for Clinical Audit, and there is considerable zeal among some of our members to make sure it works. That is how far we have come.

Macara points out that the BMA saw the tactical necessity to get on board the audit initiative: 'Of course the motivation for all of this was not entirely un-self-interested. After Griffiths it was clear management was coming in and that there was to be more measurement of performance. Doctors thought "with managers taking over we have to make sure we're keeping our end up"'.

But Macara dismisses the idea of outcomes. 'There is an air of the witch hunt about them,' he says.

People want to build outcomes up into league tables comparing performance of hospitals and surgeons. I can't agree to it, it would be difficult to put into practice, the basis for fair calculations would be very hard to draw up, and there would be errors that could wreck careers. I have seen a great change in the medical profession over the last few years, and this could jeopardise all that.

On top of the problem of defining the quality of the treatment delivered by surgeons is the question of the kind of patients they were treating. Clearly there is a considerable difference between a surgeon who sees a grievously ill elderly person go into long-term decline after an operation before dying and one who operates on a relatively young and fit person and makes him immobile and ill for the rest of his life. We must be aware of the kinds of operations doctors are carrying out if we are to judge them effectively.

The last problem is: who are we to show all this information to if we can gather it in the first place? Dr Macara says: 'I simply don't think you can make all sorts of details about doctors' activity available to the general public.' For all the above reasons he believes the data would be either too complex to understand or reduced to a simplicity which made it meaningless, misleading and dangerous. 'You can't reduce everything down to a number like a QALY', he says. 'It is too complex.'

In an ideal world, admits Dr Macara, if all the information was made available to a well-informed public, there may be a chance of seeing outcomes measurements work. That, however, is not the world we live in, he says.[17]

Macara's views are backed up by the Department of Epidemiology at the University of Dundee. According to researchers there, the casemix question is too complex to admit easy or speedy solutions and the whole philosophy of outcomes measurements sets the profession and managers on a collision course that is difficult, if not impossible, to avoid or resolve. Better, in their view, to concentrate on how treatments are administered, rather than feeding an obsession with outcomes.[18]

Still, many believe that the refusal of doctors to participate in outcomes measurement undermines the whole point of audit and measuring their activities. There is no point, they say, in measuring a process, unless we can tell whether that process does any good.

Problems of quality

Macara's objections on all these points are serious and indicate considerable practical difficulties in drawing up this kind of information. The first problem is whether we can produce meaningful information about the quality of care. Quality is a problematic and elusive word in the context of health care. Measuring the quality outcome of a treatment on an individual person is extremely complex. Death is not the only outcome. If the patient survives, there will be changes in the quality of life.

There have been a number of attempts to quantify quality of care. It can be judged, for example by the King's Fund's five point procedure. For quality health care, treatment must be appropriate, in that it is needed by the patient; the distribution of services must be equitable (available to all); the services must be accessible; resources must not be wasted; the service must satisfy the expectations of the patient, within reasonable limits, and it must be effective.[19] But as one analyst points out, there are serious contradictions between these criteria, which can leave difficult decisions on trade offs between them.

Understanding requirements and expectation of patients, sharing information and promoting learning within health organizations and setting up performance measurement techniques are crucial if the patient and the patient's interests are going to be drawn into any of these definitions. Only after these kinds of ground rules have been established can any judgements about the quality of a service be made.

Quality of life is one of the most complex areas of the quality debate. Measuring the impact on the quality of life of a given patient undergoing a given treatment depends on understanding what was expected of the treatment in the first place and measuring up the outcome to those expectations. But how? Mortality statistics are too crude. Measuring morbidity – suffering or being diseased – is much more difficult as we shall see in Chapter 9.

National Confidential Enquiry into Perioperative Deaths (NCEPOD)

There is one place where outcomes data are collected: the annual National Confidential Enquiry into Perioperative Deaths. It is the confidential bit that worries people like Alan Maynard. It also worries Brendan Devlin, the man behind its production.

Devlin has worked since 1982 on clinical audit, and has earned the suspicion of his colleagues for his efforts. Nevertheless he sees clinical audit as a crucial element of the future profession and health service. 'I would very much hope the confidential will be taken off the NCEPOD before the end of my lifetime. Unfortunately hope is the right word. There is no guarantee', he says.

The importance of publishing data, in Devlin's view, is as much to advertise the achievements of surgery as it is to show up those who are poor, even dangerous, practitioners. He believes league tables for surgeons are a long way off but there are important steps that need to be taken to make sure that the day will arrive when performance tables that measure information accurately can be used responsibly.

'I have no objection to them in principle', he says. 'The problem is, if I advocated them now I would lose the support of the medical profession for the other work I do – like NCEPOD – which is very important.'

The reason we are so far off having meaningful league tables comes back to a familiar problem – information:

> We urgently need a well informed data set so that we can see what is happening around the country. At the moment information about patients in the service is recorded as 'Finished Consultant Episodes'. These record each separate procedure that is carried out on an individual patient. So if he comes in for a hernia and has that operated on that is one thing. If he then goes to a ward and then has to be operated on again, that is recorded as another. You cannot tell from the records that it is the same patient.

> For example, the commonest cause of death in the records is through tracheotomy – making a hole in the throat to breathe - which is routinely carried out after a road accident. But because of the way data is recorded, patients are said to have died after tracheotomy rather than after a road accident.

Devlin believes that if a data set were compiled league tables, or at least meaningful outcome data could be made available to managers or GPs. In the meantime, he proposes that more information is published about surgeons – what their qualifications are, whether they have a merit award, what level the award is and so on.

The complexities of casemix are another barrier. Devlin does not see this as insurmountable. 'The BMA's objections sound like special pleading to me, and I think their objections must be overruled. They argue that it is too complicated and therefore should not be attempted. I say we should get started', says Devlin.

Devlin has found the information deficit has thwarted much of his work on NCEPOD. Early NCEPOD enquiries found 'important differences in clinical practice' between the three regions it studied. The 1992–93 NCEPOD enquiry found 'a substantial shortfall in critical care services' and recommended that 'the medical profession needs to develop and enforce standards of practice for the management of many common acute conditions, e.g. head injuries, aortic aneurysm, colorectal cancer, gastrointestinal bleeding'. 'The frequency of "lost notes" continues to be a problem both for clinicians and managers. Non-availability of notes was the stated reason for inability to return 22% of the surgical questionnaires (sent out by NCEPOD to measure deaths after operations) and 36% of anaesthetic questionnaires.' Even where notes were available they were not always of good quality.

Devlin himself says:

> We often find that something like 50% of the notes made after opera-
> tions which record how it was conducted and log the outcome don't
> have the surgeons' names, and 50% don't have the actual operation on
> them. In 1993, 77% of surgeons had entered their names but only 49.2%
> of patient notes included the diagnosis. If you can't find out how much
> work is being done and who is doing it you can't come up with any
> meaningful analysis.

The survey confirms that the name of the consultant in charge of the operation was only recorded in 56% of cases.

Devlin's work on NCEPOD has earned him little thanks from the profession:

> I had a tough time starting it. It was very intimidating. If they don't
> want to do something they can make your life very difficult, particu-
> larly as in the medical profession you are often dependent on your
> peers for promotion, status and prestige.
>   The usual argument I hear is 'we don't have enough time to audit,
> we're too busy and overwhelmed by work.' My response is often 'you
> are the only surgeon in this hospital who won't do it. I'm going to
> publish your name unless you do.'[20]

Interestingly, despite his fears about intimidation and being isolated by his peers, Devlin has an A+ merit award – the highest and rarest honour that can be bestowed on one colleague by another.

Devlin's work on NCEPOD is admired by Alan Maynard. He believes the enquiry should be brought out of the wings and into mainstream NHS practice. He argues that purchasers should require providers to include all their surgeons and anaesthetists in the NCEPOD programme, and should monitor the data as a condition of contracting with them. He also believes that the Audit Commission should be put in charge of NCEPOD, instructing NHS auditors not to endorse trust and purchaser accounts if they fail to monitor the NCEPOD performance, and says patients' recovery should be monitored to try to explain variation in rates.[21]

Box 8.1: Stitching up the surgeons

In some cases purchasers are getting in among the doctors and finding out about performance, building their knowledge about who does what best into their planning. Dr Harry Burns is a poacher turned gamekeeper – a former consultant general surgeon, he moved into public health management on the Greater Glasgow Health Board because he felt doctors and hospitals were operating without regard for how the health system worked as a whole. He wanted to take a more strategic role in the future of the health system.

Dr Burns believes measuring outcomes and using evidence-based care is crucial to the future of the system, but he believes a sensitive and responsible attitude has to be taken in order to make sure information is used and interpreted properly, and doctors are not alienated. He believes data on performance and outcomes of individual doctors should be made available, but not to the public. 'You can actually significantly mislead people, because of the complexities of case mix and the role of chance,' he says. Nevertheless, Dr Burns has used information on outcomes in Glasgow.

He started with breast cancer, where his research showed major variations in survival between surgeons. 'We got the figures for five hospitals in Glasgow on the survival of patients after surgery. The figures were surgeon specific. We then approached the surgeons and told them we had the information. We said: 'Look, we can do this the hard way or the easy way. We can make these figures public and let the public choose where they want to be treated. Or we can do it the easy way, where we decide what is effective treatment and you undertake to treat people in these ways, as set out in protocols.'

Since then Dr Burns and his team have compared performance year-on-year. They have also expanded the process across a range of other conditions, including head and neck and colorectal cancers. 'We're saying this can't be swept under the carpet any more. We are being pragmatic – we don't want to seem like Big Brother. But we are saying we want change. This is a game of carrots and sticks. The carrot is not using the stick. Professions need to have the confidence of the public to maintain the power they have. What we said initially when we did the work with the breast cancer surgeons played directly on this fact: we said the easy way is for you to change and do this, and that will preserve your professional dignity. The other way is to go public. And they are not going to stand for you or us or anyone else messing around with their lives.'

In fact doctors come round to it after initial fears. 'The initial meeting we had on the breast cancer figures will stay in my memory for a long time. The clinicians from the five hospitals came into the meeting not knowing what the outcomes were going to be. I had said we wanted consensus for change to come out of the meeting. They were deeply suspicious of each other and of my motives when the meeting started. But after the figures were presented we moved quickly from suspicion to consensus. When they were out in the open it was clear the priority was finding a way to move forward.'

Dr Burns realizes he was in a unique position to engineer the changes, having been a surgeon with a detailed knowledge of the problems he was dealing with. But he believes his experience shows that outcomes measurements can, in principle, be used to inform decisions on purchasing. He sees it as a crucial step forward in managing health services. The other side of the coin is evidence-based medicine. Dr Burns falls in line with the view of Professor David Sackett – that EBM must be built around consensus. He believes the claims that 80% of treatment is not proven to be effective are exaggerated. The issue is more about standards of proof and whether randomized controlled trial, the gold standard, is the only way to be confident that treatments are effective, and therefore worth the money spent on them.

The evidence culture needs to come into management systems to ensure that these discoveries are disseminated and put into practice. The problem is that management systems are not widespread and often not up to the task. As one study says: 'A major and widely acknowledged weakness of most health care systems is their inability to produce valid and comprehensive measures of outcome of the care provided.'[22]

Again Dr Burns's expertise is the exception that proves the rule. A survey of 15 health authorities in the West Midlands into bringing the guidelines into medical practice found: 'Guidelines development is at a very early stage and there are many pitfalls to overcome. Development is likely to be slow with much resistance along the way. Though the potential is not promising,

> the movement is justified both by the need to provide appropriate care and the promise it offers for continuing medical education.' It points out that guidelines are not easy to prepare; that they must be able to be audited; that they must have sufficient evidence to back them up; and that clinicians locally must feel they have a significant input into drawing them up – this can lead to problems over the quality of the guidelines, which tend to gravitate towards the 'lowest common denominator'. Making sure clinicians board the ship and stay on board is difficult, as are guidelines covering a variety of care groups – involving GPs and consultants.[10]
>
> Interview with Harry Burns, August 1996.

Professional roles and training

If your daughter is to benefit from the seamless system of care in 2048, and if she is to rely on care that is effective and of high quality, there will have to be major changes in the way the medical profession, nursing and support workers in the health system are organized. As we charted through Chapters 2 and 3, and as we have seen from the arguments of Cochrane, health care has been constructed on a medical model, dominated by the medical profession. That needs to change.

There are several issues: ensuring efficiency and quality through the spread of manpower, bringing effectiveness and evidence into the workplace and ensuring quality in the different places of work. The barriers to change are summed up in the words 'consultant', 'registrar', 'house officer', 'nurse', and so on. The strict labelling and compartmentalization through training and role segregation has restricted the health system every bit as much as the inflexible spine of hospitals inherited from 1962.

The problems of inflexibility

According to one study on the medical workforce:

> The professional structures of the NHS tend to have a limiting effect on the exercise of the knowledge and skills of staff. There are plenty of examples of staff not being used to the full. A recent example to hit the headlines is the shortage of senior house officers in Accident and

Emergency (A&E). This shortage would not have such major implications if nursing roles in A&E had been expanded to include a significant amount of the junior medical workload. The reality in many A&E departments is that senior nurses play an active, although unrecognized, role in the training and supervision of junior doctors.[23]

The role of nursing

As traditional demarcations have continued in the teeth of strong pressures for change, the working lives of health professionals have become less attractive. Nursing has become an undesirable occupation instead of a vocation. The number of pre-registration nursing students has dropped from 87 570 in 1983 to 58 131 in 1995 – a fall of a third. This fall has occurred at a time when the skills of nurses are in demand as never before and as future strategies for a primary care-led system will require more from them.[24]

When nurses hit the headlines it is often to do with pay. The Royal College of Nursing (RCN) spends much of its campaigning time concentrating on pay disputes – particularly after local pay was brought in. This has not noticeably affected hospital doctors, but nurses claim they have been hit by derisory rises from the centre that have not been matched by the promised top-ups locally. They are also often employed on short-term contracts. While doctors have the autonomy noted in Chapter 2, nurses suffer low pay and low security. This can only serve to underline traditional divisions within the health workforce, giving nurses the view that they are undervalued.

Much has been written about the need for a primary care-led NHS with a primary care team capable of delivering it. Yet, according to the RCN, community nurses are not fully integrated into primary care by GPs. Neither is their newly-won permission to prescribe being encouraged around the country. At the same time the number of community nurses has been cut.

Public attitudes limit the speed of change. Medical organizations are loathe to give up their professional status and so stories of nurses carrying out inappropriate tasks are frequently leaked to the media. Opposition to more flexible 'generic carers' is unanimous among professional groups and unions.[25]

Manpower difficulties

There are not enough doctors in Britain. Training requirements and the length of courses has traditionally kept numbers low, which has limited the flexibility of the medical profession. In acute specialties, public health and general practice there were a total of 72 552 in England and Wales. The need to change training methods to allow more doctors – particularly consultants – has been recognized by a report from the Chief Medical Officer Sir Kenneth Calman. The report recommended the amalgamation of four of the medical training grades into two to allow a greater inflow of trained specialists.[26]

A recent report by the Senate of Surgery of the Royal College of Surgeons recognized that there were still problems and pressures for change. It pointed to rising patient expectations, the need for increased specialization to improve outcomes, new technology and reduction in junior doctors' hours, which all required a change in the way training was organized, and in how staffing patterns were arranged. In addition, recent reports have indicated alarming lapses in training and supervision of junior doctors by consultant staff.[27]

One of the key problems was the district general hospital (DGH) itself. We have seen the problems of inflexibility that the network of DGHs has presented to service co-ordinators and purchasers in the last chapter. The Senate believes the pressures for change demand that a more strategic and flexible view of how services are provided be taken. It recommends specifically that service planning moves from looking to cover populations of 200 000 to 250 000, and looks instead at populations from 450 000 to 500 000. This would be possible with better management, organization of training, and technology, and would allow the already stretched profession to increase the quality and efficiency with which it delivers services.[28]

An evidence-based profession

The problems of clinical training and staffing are not driven purely, or even primarily, by logistical pressures. The very culture of the service – the training methods articulated by Cochrane – limit its ability to meet the needs of the patients it serves.

Methods of training are still what Sir Michael Peckham would term 'empirical', despite the fact that studies are showing that evidence-based training can lead to better outcomes. As one analyst concluded, clinical guidelines, if incorporated into medical training and practice, can lead to higher quality.[29]

In addition, the segregation of professional roles has led to inhibited quality and 'problem solving'. One study counsels that: 'Doctors and nurses working together in health care teams must move away from responses in solving clinical problems to formulate those problems in a series of answerable questions.' This involves incorporating evidence and guidelines into practice using the skills both of doctors and nurses.

The study continued:

> Such a move to evidence-based health care is intellectually and economically appealing but requires the erosion of the model in which doctors develop guidelines while nurses and therapists carry them out. There is a need to accept that nurses will end up leading doctors in many areas – for example cardiac rehabilitation, incontinence and palliative care. The need for professional integration was even greater in primary care, where hospital doctors traditionally did most research and passed it onto GPs. Now nurses, GPs and hospital doctors must work together.[30]

The profession recognizes the need for change and some want it for themselves. Starting at the grass roots, the profession is asking itself what it wants out of professional life. One GP argues that changes in the speed and quality of information in concert with social values – focusing more on community concerns – will drive doctors towards wanting greater flexibility, dynamism, education and risk in their professional lives:

> The future will look less clear-cut, and many options will open up. Risk taking will seem more acceptable, and career changes and career breaks will appear as enticing opportunities, rather than as threats to future professional success. The shift in thinking may have fundamental implications for medical workforce planning.[31]

New working patterns are already coming to pass. According to another GP the changes in the relationship between GPs and the health system that the reform has tended to point towards the future are actually coming to pass now. Traditional contracting structures – individual agreements between GPs and health authorities – may be the norm and may continue to be so for the immediate future, but fundholding has introduced the concept of a two-way contract, with the practice providing services as well as commissioning or purchasing care from the hospital sector. Practices could become more autonomous, having a greater say in the commissioning and provision of services for populations – as in the commissioning models that we have examined elsewhere.[32]

Lastly comes a development that brings the debate about the contractual status of the doctor back full circle to the foundation of the NHS: the salaried doctor as employee of trust or health authority. Pilots in Liverpool and Newcastle have broken the taboo, and show how general practice can be offered as a clinical service alongside traditional, hospital-based services. This points to a breakdown in the boundaries between primary and secondary care. The breakdown could be greatly constructive for the future – allowing greater initiative and co-operation between doctors. After a period when GPs, consultants and managers have been at each others' throats, more flexible and community-focused practice could lead to a reinvigoration of the profession itself.

While there are positive implications, it is important not to discard the lessons of that period of conflict – particularly that there is value in separating purchasing/commissioning of care from provision. General practice is one area where the split has been corrupted, and the models outlined above could entrench this breach, downplaying the need for financial rigour. It is essential that control of costs accompanies new flexible formats if the system is to operate with any hope of future sustainability. Health authorities may have to take a strategic 'purchaser' view of the activities going on beneath it in the arenas formerly known as primary and secondary care.

Towards the future: quality throughout the system

The problems of compartmentalized professions are well known across industry, and moves to break down traditional barriers have resulted in greater efficiency and quality across the spectrum of organizations. The NHS is lagging.

Conroy et al. characterize the health workforce as fragmented and locked into traditional profiles. The fragmentation has problems for the accountability of the profession as we noted in Chapter 3. It also wastes time and limits flexibility. But Conroy believes the forces for change will create a better-functioning organization. 'The opportunity is there to create new roles which would be more challenging and fulfilling for staff whilst at the same time providing benefits in terms of the quality, continuity and cost-effectiveness of services.'[23]

His study points to wider use of 'generic carers' and 'support workers' to help re-model services. Generic carers would deliver most care, with responsibility for co-ordinating the service across disciplines. The generic carer – a 'super nurse' – would take over many of the responsibilities of doctors, who would focus on highly specialist procedures. In addition, the number of technicians will drop.

This new scenario would have a number of benefits: the workforce would be more focused on patient needs, there would be greater flexibility and quality as well as job satisfaction for workers. The service would begin to remodel itself for the new millennium.[23]

Labour

The Government has stated its support for EBM and for the necessity to ensure clinical effectiveness is at the forefront of policy. It has set up the National Institute for Clinical Excellence to 'give new coherence and prominence to information about clinical and cost effectiveness'.[33] This could prove to be a powerful force for change. It has also launched a series of clinical indicators that are intended to lever measurement of quality into the hospital league tables. The proposals are for 15 indicators measuring such factors as death in hospital within 30 days of surgery, emergency admissions within 28 days of previous discharge, surgery for recurrence of hernia and damage to organs in hospital following an operation.[34]

The introduction of the measures was welcomed by Sir Norman Bowse, Chairman of the BMA Joint Consultant's Committee, which will work together with the Government in drawing up, testing and integrating the quality indicators into existing hospital league tables.

These initiatives are a significant development and could introduce both real quality measurement into the system as well as producing genuinely meaningful accountability. Time will tell whether it goes the way of clinical audit or whether it could breathe new life into the old initiative.

References

1 Cochrane A (1971) *Effectiveness and Efficiency: random reflections on health services*. Nuffield Provincial Hospitals Trust, London.
2 Timmins N (1996) NHS 'wastes £1bn on ineffective measures'. *Independent*. 2 January.
3 Interview with Dr Sandy Macara, July 1996.
4 *Table manners at the health care feast: the case for spending less and getting more from the NHS*, speech by Alan Maynard at London School of Economics, 26 October 1995.
5 Bevan G and Devlin HB (1995) *Medical Practice Variation*. Social Market Foundation, London.
6 Appleby J, Walshe K and Ham C (1995) *Acting on the Evidence*. NAHAT, Birmingham.
7 NHS Executive (1996) *Promoting Clinical Effectiveness*. NHSE, London.
8 Interview with Sir Michael Peckham, July 1996.
9 Sackett D (1996) Evidence-based Medicine: what it is and what it isn't. *BMJ*. 312: 71–2.
10 Honigsbaum F and Ham C (1996) *Improving Clinical Effectiveness: the develop-*

ment of clinical guidelines in the West Midlands. University of Birmingham, Birmingham.

11 Ham C (1992) *Health Policy in Britain*. (3rd ed.) Macmillan, Basingstoke.

12 DoH (1989) *Working for Patients* (Cmnd 555). HMSO, London.

13 Klein R (1995) *The New Politics of the National Health Service*. (3rd ed.) Longman, Harlow.

14 National Audit Office (1995) *Clinical Audit in England*. HMSO, London.

15 Kerrison S, Packwood T and Buxton M (1993) *Medical Audit: taking stock*. King's Fund Centre, London.

16 Spiers J (1995) *The Invisible Hospital and the Secret Garden: an insider's commentary on the NHS reforms*. Radcliffe Medical Press, Oxford.

17 Interview with Dr Sandy Macara, July 1996.

18 Davies H and Crombie I (1995) Assessing the quality of care. *BMJ*. **311**: 766–7.

19 Maxwell R (1984) Quality assessment in health. *BMJ*. **288**.

20 Interview with Brendan Devlin, July 1996; see also Campling E, Devlin HB, Hoile RW *et al.* (1995) *The Report of the National Confidential Enquiry into Perioperative Deaths 1992/93*. NCEPOD, London.

21 Maynard A (1996) Health: a matter of facts. *Health Service Journal*.

22 Donaldson L (1996) Impact of management on outcomes, in M Peckham and R Smith (eds) *Scientific Basis of Health Services*. BMJ Publishing Group, London.

23 Conroy M, Glascott F, Cochrane D *et al.* (1996) *The Future Healthcare Workforce: steering group report*. University of Manchester, Manchester, p. 77.

24 Royal College of Nursing (1996) *National Health Manifesto*. RCN, London.

25 Brindle D (1996) Nurses balk at 'generic carer' role. *Guardian*. 23 May; Timmins N (1996) Cleaners become carers in brave new world. *Independent*. 23 May.

26 Calman K (1993) *Hospital Doctors: training for the future*. Department of Health, London.

27 Audit Commission (1996) *The Doctor's Tale Continued: the audits of hospital medical staffing*. HMSO, London; Suzman M (1996) Watchdog attacks NHS training. *Financial Times*. 5 June; Mihill C (1996) Consultants 'fail to watch juniors'. *Guardian*. 5 June.

28 Senate of Surgery of Great Britain and Ireland (1997) *Consultant Surgical Practice and Training in the UK*. Senate of Surgery of Great Britain and Ireland, London.

29 Mulrow C (1996) Critical look at clinical guidelines, in M Peckham and R Smith (eds) *Scientific Basis of Health Services*. BMJ Publishing Group, London.

30 Kitson A, McManus C and Pringle M (1996) A research base for professional staffing of health services, in M Peckham and R Smith (eds) *Scientific Basis of Health Services*. BMJ Publishing Group, London.

31 Harrison J (1998) *The GP Tomorrow: living with uncertainty*. Radcliffe Medical Press, Oxford.

32 Interview with Michael Dixon, GP, Collumpton, Devon, August 1997.

33 Secretary of State for Health (1997) *The New NHS* (Cmnd 3807). HMSO, London.

34 DoH (1997) *NHS to be judged on quality, not just quantity of care*. 9 July (press release).

9 Rationing

From the day the NHS was set up and the Government took responsibility for financing the nation's health care it also took responsibility for rationing it. Attitudes to rationing have been complex and contradictory ever since. Officially, its existence is denied because of the promise that the system would universalize the best. However, acceptance that resources have to be allocated because demand always outstrips supply has worked in parallel to this. Throughout the first two decades of the system, the rationing dilemma remained where it was – submerged in the system – but as economic fortune turned downwards it became clearer, until the 1990 reforms caused many to believe the issue would be forced out into the open.

Those who lived through the war will have had different attitudes to rationing. The very word rationing suggested reason in the face of scarcity. They grew up in a world where resources were limited; people now are more demanding consumers. The consumers of the future will be even more so and, as with issues of accountability and funding, it is quite possible that they will increasingly question the competence of health bureaucracies to make decisions on health care for them. They may have to rely heavily on doctors and managers for advice, but is it really likely that the citizens of 2048 will accept being told what they can and can't have by a computer in a distant office or a doctor they have met once? Is it not more likely that they will want at least to understand, if not be involved in, the decision-making process themselves?

The issue is critical to the future of the system. As confidence in the justice of the rationing process subsides, so too does the legitimacy of the NHS itself, but the reality is undeniable: the health system is, in fact a rationing system allocating resources by decisions taken in a bureaucracy in the absence of a price mechanism to do the job instead.

The secret tradition of rationing care

From the Cabinet table down through the health authority to the surgeon and GP, decisions about how much money should be spent on what and given to whom and when have been made since the foundation of the NHS.

Rationing has been hidden and decisions are taken by 'pluralistic bargaining between different lobbies modified by shifting political judgements made in the light of changing pressures.'[1]

Although rationing may have been considered a fair process in allocating food, it had to be kept a secret when distributing health care. Enoch Powell, Health Secretary from 1960 to 1963 explained how and why the system operated:

> The public are encouraged to believe that rationing in medical care was banished by the National Health Service, and that the very idea of rationing being applied to medical care is immoral and repugnant. Consequently when they, and the medical profession too, come face to face in practice with the various forms of rationing to which the National Health Service must resort, the usual result is bewilderment, frustration and irritation.

As this point makes clear, it was not an easy truce between doctors and politicians.[2]

As we have seen, GPs vary in their referral patterns, and in their prescribing and treatment habits. The same variations are true of consultants, who have personal views on the effectiveness of specific treatments and who apply hospital 'queuing' systems in different ways. Consultants may ration services in a number of ways that would be criticized if they were adopted into mainstream 'priority setting' practice. For example, they may ration according to age – the case of setting an age limit for the provision of expensive dialysis treatment for elderly sufferers of kidney disease. Hospital doctors' own values may play an important part in deciding whether to offer cancer treatment to smokers. Again such difficult ethical questions have traditionally been addressed by the individual doctor exercising individual judgements, hidden away from the limelight of the public commissioning arena.

The rationing dilemma pulls into sharp focus the tensions in the doctor's situation. The doctor is being asked to exist within parameters being set out by the health authority in the decisions it takes in prioritizing health care. Although doctors have a right to challenge the priorities because no treatment can be ruled out, this amounts to a right of veto. If budgets on treatments that lie outside agreed protocols between the trust and the health authority are too high, hospital management can make it clear to the doctor that clinical freedom can be stretched only so far. The doctor is being asked to bend clinical freedom to fit within the principles of equity, justice and utility that management demands. In other words clinical freedom and medical individualism are left intact to deal with difficult situations, but must toe the line in the day-to-day running of services. It is a system which makes financial management difficult and causes frequent conflict.

Rationing by doctors is at one end of a complex interaction of groups and interests involved in sharing out resources. Techniques have been refined over the history of the post-war system. They have been characterized as *deterrence* (the decision of a GP or GP's administrative staff to make an appointment later rather than sooner or not at all), *delay* (through the referral procedure with its waiting lists for outpatient consultations with specialists and treatment), *dilution* (to the hospital where the decision on how and what to treat will be taken), before, finally, the *decision* on how long to keep a patient in hospital is taken – and *termination of treatment*.[1]

The decision-making problems flowing through the system are hedged around with difficulties. For the Government, the question will be: 'What is the appropriate total for the health budget?' This has a direct influence on the necessity for rationing and the extent to which services will have to be rationed. What effects will education or housing spending have on health? (A question raised by investigations into equity such as the Black Report in the 1980s, but kept away from public debate at least ever since.) Once an amount is agreed, how is it to be distributed? On what side of the service should it be spent: primary or hospital, prevention or cure? What sort of treatments should it buy – those that have been used historically, or only those with a proven scientific legitimacy? How much public involvement should there be?

Each decision taken at one level effects the boundaries within which decisions further down the chain can be taken. So if the Health Secretary extracts enough from the Cabinet discussions on major increases in the budget the amount of funding flowing to health authorities and GP fundholders out to the hospitals and community services to the GP as provider will consequently be greater, giving greater room for manoeuvre. Pessimists will argue that it simply allows another thin slice of the limitless mountain of demand to be included among the lucky few who are treated. The flow, however, is a complex interaction of decisions, each determined by the relationships between each group, and the philosophy guiding each group at any given time.

There is also a difference between priority setting and rationing. Priority setting, in Klein's view, is the process of deciding broad priorities – the Government's decisions about which services should receive increases in public funds, the decision of the Department of Health in setting broad policy guidelines and of health authorities in deciding how to prioritize treatments. Rationing is a term more properly used to describe what doctors do – decide which individuals shall be treated and which shall be put on a waiting list, or not be treated.

As we shall see, the distinction between broad policy and day-to-day implementation is one that will have to be used in whatever decision is taken about rationing more rationally. But the search for rationalism must accept the fundamental dilemma that Klein's attempt at clarification throws up: there is a very grey area between the broad decisions taken on principle by a Government or rationing committee of experts and the practical, pragmatic concerns dealt with by doctors every day, which may undermine the very legitimacy of any overall system.

Do we need to ration openly or at all?

There is debate, not just over how open these rationing decisions are, but about how open they should be. On the one extreme some individuals go back to the underlying controversy that has justified the rationing debate and pointed to the need for greater health authority involvement. They argue that the case for infinite demand for health care outstripping finite supply has not been conclusively settled and say the public should be asked not how we ration health care, but whether we wish to. This would shift attention to the question of whether more resources are needed in the system as a whole.[3]

At the other extreme some argue that there is a necessity to ration, but counsel against naively opening up decision making to the sorts of processes outlined here, but to continue in time honoured fashion to 'muddle through elegantly'. Thus: 'We should resist abandoning an admittedly imperfect though workable irrationality in favour of a spurious and possibly risky rationality.'[4]

The question is another taboo in British life.

Forces for change

The doctor's role

The legitimacy of rationing is under question as never before. A series of factors is at work. First there is the perceived build up in demand through demographic, expectational and technology driven factors. On top of this is the structure that the reforms have created: the split between purchaser and provider, and the focusing on the contract relationship. Third, this has called into question the traditional role of the doctor as the individual who decides who shall be treated and who shall wait. Instead attention has begun to focus on the commissioner – the health authority, GP fundholder or commissioning group.

The medical profession is in some cases becoming less willing to play its implicit rationing role any longer. Both general practitioners and hospital doctors have seen their roles change dramatically. Clinical freedom has been constrained and the pressure to manage resources for populations instead of thinking about particular patients has increased pressure on the relationship between doctors and managers.

These pressures have been most sharply focused on the GP fundholder: we saw in a previous chapter how some GPs are unwilling to take responsibility for making budgetary-enforced rationing decisions. The difficulties doctors have in rationing reflect the fact that there is strong pressure for change. Traditional relationships in the rationing system are being thrown into conflict in the opening up of health care decision making, and are themselves mutating, spurred on by the very financial alterations that are making rationing necessary.

One of the results of this is to bring the fragmentation dilemma into clear focus. It also points out the central paradox of fundholding. Despite the intense opposition that has accompanied its history, fundholding has certainly brought the awareness of the financial aspects of health care to the grass roots of the service. It has brought the GP into the health care commissioning process. However, while making people aware of what is needed it has remained incapable of delivering it. If one accepts that fundholding has fragmentary tendencies then it follows that taking a strategic, commissioning view, is difficult, if not impossible. Fragmentation is also likely to undermine equity because decisions are not taken against a strategic background that attempts to guarantee a standard of care for all. So the fragmenting tendency of fundholding fragments rationing decisions too.

Health authorities setting priorities in purchasing plans are seen as an assault on the freedom of individual doctors to make decisions themselves. Deciding between treatment at district level therefore limits the freedom of the doctor to act in the patients' best interests. Making these pressures more explicit exacerbates the situation, rendering doctors less able to exercise clinical judgement and be flexible.

One said: 'I can see the point of not doing things which are ineffective. But we must be able to decide ourselves what is and what is not. There can be guidelines, but in the final analysis, it must be us who make the decision.'[5]

So, the contribution of the medical profession to resolving difficult dilemmas is reinforced by its insistence on clinical freedom. As Sir Duncan Nichol suggests, the more that freedom is threatened, the less likely doctors are to co-operate and 'do the dirty work'. The hospital doctor exists in a wider context of priority setting.[6]

The health authority

The second change is the splitting off of the purchasing function, which has made those pressures more open. In the case of the fundholding GP this may or may not be welcome. In the case of the hospital doctor, the methods of rationing will change as the range of treatments is prescribed by purchasers – as an explicit form of rationing. Instead of the traditional arrangement where doctors take decisions within ill-defined boundaries created by other players in the system, the purchasers themselves are becoming more bound up with actual rationing decisions. In some cases they are explicitly saying 'no', or getting as near to saying 'no' as possible, rather than drawing up interpretable priorities and handing the tough decisions over to doctors.

Logically, these pressures point towards a greater role for health authorities. In their purchasing role there is a great deal of scope for defining those treatments they will and will not pay for, for taking decisions openly, rationally and with legitimacy in the minds of patients and the public. The health authority occupies a strategic position. And as Harrison and Hunter point out, central government seeks to avoid difficulties over rationing by diffusing decision making to the local level. However, reality is slow to catch up with logic.[7]

Health authorities, like GP fundholders, are recognizing their new roles in the process, and embracing them with different levels of enthusiasm.

According to studies made by a team at Bath University, the use of explicit rationing is, on one level, becoming more widespread: while 11 authorities listed treatments they would exclude in 1994–95, the number had climbed to 23 in 1995–96 and 26 in 1996–97. Since the reforms there has been a move towards these kinds of decisions, but it has been slow.[8]

The study also indicates that change in purchasing plans is incremental, and thus that historical decisions on prioritizing for treatment are built into today's purchasing plans. These factors are probably far more influential than high-profile explicit exclusions – they are very difficult to measure.

Although purchasing plans are not allowed by Government explicitly to rule out treatments, health authorities effectively try to do so. The reality remains that health authorities can use the conventions of clinical freedom to pass the buck, claiming that doctors must interpret the broad outlines of their policies in their day-to-day work. Thus they allow doctors clinical freedom, and they pass the hard questions – is x treatment (low funding priority) justifiable in the case of y patient (65, with recurring condition)? – while effectively constricting them. The grey area persists.

Box 9.1: Buckinghamshire Health Authority

In June 1997, Buckinghamshire Health Authority sent out a leaflet explaining that it had to recoup a £4 million overspend on the previous year caused by meeting Patient's Charter standards, increased demand for mental health and A&E services and a rise in drug costs. In order to keep A&E services it declared that: 'Patients with the greatest medical need are being given priority for treatment. This means that care for some people may no longer be available through the NHS or that waiting times for treatment will increase.' Services affected included chiropody, schools health services, family planning, community dentistry, and speech and language therapy. It added a section on what it termed 'low priority treatments' stating that its criteria for judging would be effectiveness. Low priority treatments on this criterion included cosmetic surgery, homeopathy and IVF – services which the health authority did not buy.

Equity

One in six authorities now effectively excludes certain treatments from NHS provision – treatments such as cosmetic surgery, tattoo removal, sex change and renal dialysis for over 65s. In more contentious cases such as IVF there are different levels of provision depending on where you live. In some parts of Britain it is free; in Somerset you pay £500–£1500 per treatment. In Liverpool treatment goes only to those under 35; in Humberside to those under 40.

At health authority level there are a number of questions. It is not only straight and explicit rationing that has implications for equity. Although these implications will be strong (why should patients in Northamptonshire not be able to get IVF while a woman in Birmingham is given help by the NHS in a vain attempt to have octuplets?) there are other important problems of equity involving purchasers.

In some cases the development of services that are deemed to be too expensive will be shelved, postponed or not considered. This has clear implications for the comparability of services between districts nearby and further afield. Multiple sclerosis sufferers may find they live in an area like North and Mid Hampshire which has decided against funding beta interferon, while patients in other parts of the country may have access to the experimental drug.

Health authorities may argue they should not fund experimental treatments as that is effectively subsidising private sector R&D programmes. But this is at best simply shifting the cost – the increased R&D cost will come back as increased price and must be funded by someone whether fundholder health authority or commissioning group. The logic overall is that purchasing/commissioning should become more responsive to community needs and more influential in deciding how to spend budgets. It gains legitimacy and power that way.

The point is that one man's expression of the individual preferences of a community expressed through its commissioning group is another's fragmentation. From the reforming viewpoint, increased emphasis on choice not only accepts that there are differences in level and quality of provision around the country, but uses this as a justification for policy. But this conviction – which underpins the choice-based market – is not carried through consistently. There is an acceptance that such logic must exist, within perception at least, that the system is national and equitable.

Public consultation

Health authorities may include other criteria for making decisions that increase their legitimacy. Some, like West Glamorgan Health Authority, have set up advisory committees on the ethics of rationing. Similar groups have been set up by fundholding GPs.[1,4,7,9]

There are problems with public consultation. According to one study – which claims to be the first prioritization exercise of a random sample of a national population – those surveys of local populations that do exist show public priorities favour acute treatments over preventative treatments and those for chronic illnesses.[10]

If the public is forced to take decisions, it is likely to want to make 'easier' decisions on which new demands on resources should be met, rather than deciding which of a number of treatments should be cut. Likewise, the value-laden nature of decisions, and the likelihood that these will be more prevalent in the public mind in the case of specific groups of the population – defined by age, or behaviour – than they will be in specific treatments, may influence decisions towards defining on whom money should be spent rather than on what. Those treatments on which the public feels it can come to an agreement may be relatively uncontentious – like tattoo removal or nose surgery – and may not, as we have noted before, be effective rationing.

What is an illness?

Rationing decisions have traditionally been taken in a number of ways that are not clearly explained. There is rationing by exclusion, identifying certain treatments that will not be supplied – like, for example spa treatment – available in (more expensive) European health services but not on the NHS. Other examples might be minor treatments like removal of varicose veins or tattoos. As the reforms have made the tensions to define these treatments greater, the categorization of treatments such as IVF as 'low priority' and therefore, in the words of one health authority, 'something the individual should be responsible for themselves' has grown.

The basis on which these decisions are made is mixed and unclear. Sometimes there is simply no explanation of why a treatment is being excluded. Others suggest that a particular form of treatment is not something the NHS should be providing. This implies that the NHS makes a decision on what kind of condition ought to be classified as worthy of care. Infertility, for example, is classified as a legitimate condition in some areas, and not in others. This addresses fundamental social values. Is having children within the aim of the NHS? Does having them promote the serenity in society it was designed to create – if promoting that serenity is still an explicit aim of the system? Ought one to have the right to have children? Have values changed over time so that our view of the family and the importance of children in today's dynamic society is different from in the past? Does technology and the costs it brings with it – IVF is very expensive – force us to be more critical of our values?

Authorities excluding IVF give a number of reasons for doing so – Hertfordshire, Redbridge and Waltham Forest and Northamptonshire all question its effectiveness and cost effectiveness – but other authorities are concerned about whether it is a suitable condition for the NHS to treat. Some authorities introduce questions that themselves betray a set of value judgements about the way in which children relate to society – for example, requiring that couples need to have a stable relationship to qualify.

Effectiveness

Other analysts have recognized the intention to apply evidence-based medicine as a way of taking difficult decisions on allocating resources by funding only such treatments as can be proven to be effective. This will give a legitimacy to such decisions, changing the perception of them as rationing decisions – which are considered unpopular, irrational, arbitrary and unfair – to priority setting decisions, which are seen as necessary, rational and fairer. On the face of it, this is a sensible policy that should be the foundation for any rationing policy.

The trend towards using effectiveness criteria has grown – grommets and glue ear are common among exclusions. Sir Michael Peckham, director of research and development for the department of health says: 'I have always thought that the system of allocating care is arbitrary now, given the lack of evidence-based care today.' He says that the deep problems of rationing may not be solved but could be eased by the application of evidence-based medicine – allowing only those treatments that were proven to be effective to be made available, stopping the waste on those which are not.[11]

It is not quite as simple as that. The treatments mentioned above are not massive drains on the NHS purse. Effectiveness can be used as a criterion for rationing more easily in some cases than in others. What is ineffective for 99% of people may be effective for one in a hundred. Should that treatment therefore be excluded? Perversely, clinical effectiveness may lead back to the scientific rationalism which underpinned acceptance of the post-war system, at the same time proving that that system was neither scientific nor rational.

Cost effectiveness

There are difficulties of coming up with a method of converting evidence-based medicine into evidence-based rationing. Given the level of controversy surrounding marginal treatments, and the difficulty with which evidence-based protocols and guidelines are being drawn up, accepted and used in the health service, these are considerable objections.

There are various methods for putting cost effectiveness into practice. One is the quality adjusted life year (QALY). This is a measurement calculated by using medical research to match treatments to conditions to work out their precise effects on different patients. The effect of the treatment is then converted into an expected effect on the length and quality of the patient's life – coming up with a figure, known as the QALY. The total cost of the treatment is then divided by the number of QALYs it is judged to produce, giving a figure by which treatments can be ranked. So, for example, GP advice to stop smoking is cheap, and if heeded has a very positive impact on health and quality of life. It therefore has a low cost per QALY – on one calculation 167. Blood dialysis, on the other hand is a very expensive and intrusive treatment with serious implications for quality of life and limited effectiveness. It therefore has a very high cost per QALY (14 000). (The aim of QALYs would be to rank all treatments and then use them to maximize the health gain within any given health system's budget.)[7,12]

These techniques are highly controversial. A hip replacement has a lower cost per QALY than a heart transplant but does that really mean we must limit or strike off heart transplants in the event of money being scarce? Methodological difficulties and the problems of differing patients work against such systems, which would just be 'grinding out' mechanical decisions. They could also be seen as remote, an attempt by decision makers to avoid having to make decisions, clothing them instead in a spurious technological legitimacy.

Such a mechanistic approach has foundered in those parts of the world where it has been tried – for example in Oregon, where progress in implementing such a policy, started in 1989, has been very slow indeed. It was beset by difficulties such as anomalies thrown up by the calculation process, leading to the framework being changed several times. There were data deficiencies and public consultation was of questionable value.[13]

The rescue principle

In addition to these methodological difficulties, the purchaser has to take into account another variable: public opinion. Health authorities have, as we have seen, been squeezed into the rationing role by pressures from below and above – from doctors and politicians. Public sentiment may limit their alternatives further. The 'serenity' that is woven into the fabric of assumptions that justify our public health system may be better served by other conditions. The result may be that the public reaction is fierce towards decisions taken using efficiency criteria. The notion that all resources should be thrown at someone who has a disease, even if the likelihood of health gain and cost benefit are very low – known as the rescue principle – may be strong.

Thus, in the case of 'Child B' when a health authority refused to buy treatment for a child suffering from leukaemia on the grounds that it was not likely to work, there was a public outcry. The case paraded the kind of rationing decisions being made by health authorities in the public arena in a way that was without precedent. Behind the emotional headlines – 'Sentenced to Death' was typical – the harrowing issue was the decision of the health authority not to pay for chemotherapy and a bone marrow transplant after similar treatment had already failed to work. The health authority said treatment would cause great trauma without a great chance of success. When a doctor who had advised Child B's father argued that there was a 20% chance of success – much higher than had previously been suggested – the health authority still refused to pay. Circumstances took another twist when an anonymous donor paid for the treatment, which at first seemed successful. But in May 1996 Child B (real name Jaymee Bowen) died.[14]

The case illustrates how rationing decisions must resolve tensions between the individual and the wider public. On the one hand Jaymee's father argues his daughter was entitled to the treatment. But it was doctors, taking the individual's view into account, who had firstly said that the pain and trauma would not justify the treatment. It was the second doctor who argued that treatment would be worth trying, and on whose evidence Jaymee's father made a vain attempt through the Court of Appeal to have the health authority's decision overturned. The health authority looked after the interests of the public at large, whose resources should be used most effectively – and decided to take the advice of the first set of doctors.

The conflict was between those, on the one hand, who argued that patients had the right to expect a doctor to act in their interests and for the health system to comply. On the other hand the health authority argued that resources had to be allocated to those whom they were most likely to benefit.

The processes hitherto have been unclear. But as the body of evidence-based guidelines grows, some health authorities are discovering that they can make more decisions on the basis of their findings. It is, however, unclear whether this will reinforce decisions already made or whether it will be used to alter them. These forms of rationing can be the results of value judgements or calculations using the techniques of effectiveness, cost effectiveness and cost utility or both.[15]

Deciding between people

The Jaymee Bowen case involved decisions about whether an individual can benefit from treatment. There have been a number of other instances of rationing where questions about the individual are asked before treatment is given which have nothing to do with the extent of illness or the capacity to benefit from treatment.

We can ration by age. The exclusion of elderly people from renal dialysis is a commonly cited example. Justification is on economic grounds, saying that resources should be spent on younger people, who could benefit more. The opposing argument is that elderly people have paid into the NHS for many years.

Value judgements can be made about individuals. Do they have dependants? Are they economically active? Do they contribute to society? Are they poor, and therefore victims of inequity? Do they smoke, eat unhealthily, engage in dangerous sports? All of these can be used as criteria for making rationing decisions. But, like applying a perception of family values to IVF, they can be construed as unjust and arbitrary.

Rational rationing

There is little doubt that rationing has become more of an issue after reform. But Powell's law still applies. Just as there is increasing pressure to bring rationing into the open, opposition to doing so is as strong as ever.

Box 9.2: Stephen Dorrell

A previous Health Secretary, Stephen Dorrell, has claimed to confront rationing problems head on. Last year he said 'success depends on the continued willingness of the NHS to face difficult decisions about health care priorities.' He added: 'No society, in this or any other country, has the ability to provide every treatment that patients would wish. Recognition of this basic fact requires us to face difficult decisions.' He went on to anatomize the decision-making structure in the NHS – Ministers setting a framework for national priorities, purchasers assessing the needs of the people in their areas, and clinicians who 'decide the most clinically appropriate priority for each patient, based on their assessment of the patient's need.' He said these decisions must be taken in the context of 'clearly defined values' – equity, efficiency and responsiveness. He added: 'The Government has also made it clear ... That there should be no clinically effective treatments which any health authority decides as a matter of principle should never be provided.'[16]

Dorrell was neither saying anything new, nor taking the system any further forward in 'facing difficult decisions'. His statement was riddled with the loopholes that have characterized the 'explicitness' of rationing throughout the reform period. Even he, who seemed so keen to confront issues, was in fact a disperser of political heat *par excellence*.

There are two dilemmas that face policymakers, the public, the medical profession and managers: 'what is an illness?' and 'what is a doctor?' Here we review several suggestions for dealing with these issues.

Individual responsibility

Professor Ronald Dworkin is one of the world's leading experts on medical ethics. Like the advocates of a clearer private/public split noted in earlier chapters, he believes these decisions should be taken by individuals alone. In a 1996 lecture, he asked his audience to imagine an ideal world in which wealth was evenly distributed, information about medicine was freely available, people made decisions rationally, parents placed as much importance on decisions for their children as they did on decisions about themselves, and genetics were not invented. Then, he believes, the Government could keep out of providing health care, and a more just – and equitable – system would emerge. People would decide how much they would like to spend on what kind of care.

People would be unlikely, Dworkin contends, to buy an expensive policy that allowed expensive care when in a persistent vegetative state, preferring the life-support machine to be turned off. They are also more likely to buy policies that cover their children for meningitis treatment than for life-saving treatment for themselves at the age of 85. In short, the system would become clearer as to its duties and responsibilities to the specific patient in front of it because that patient would have given specific instructions to that system. This would help avoid the painful arguments over priority setting that are imposed by budget restrictions on a system where there is little scope for finding people's realistic assessment of their needs in relation to their costs.

Health care is different from other goods, and the rescue instinct is strong enough to allow money to have been spent on Jaymee Bowen to prolong her life, albeit not public money. We do not all have perfect access to perfect information; we do not always take rational decisions, income is not evenly distributed, and genetics have been discovered. So would we accept a system that told us when we were 75 that we decided when we were 40 not to have heart treatment, so unless we stumped up £15 000, there was no chance of a bypass? In this case, our life expectancy could have changed considerably in the intervening 35 years, and the thought of missing the next 35, never watching our great grandchildren pass their GCSEs and move on to university, may seem a right unfairly denied by the pressures of the system rather than by our own free choice. Would we not still blame the doctor for not making it clear we were at risk? Or the geneticist who must have been able to tell us that there was such a likelihood? Or the government for not promoting greater equality or distributing subsidies, allowing us to afford the up-to-90 policy?

In Professor Dworkin's view, it is more likely to take the form of a system – similar to the NERA prototype – where the State defines the package of care it wishes to buy, with the rest available through insurance.[17]

A right to health care

Some believe that the establishment of a general right to health care would spearhead a drive towards equity in general, within which a rationing framework could be created. The framework would allow citizens themselves to be involved, and to see their priorities reflected in whatever system is drawn up.

Some say rights should be embodied in national guidelines. The introduction of a legal right to health care should be explored, so that in the event of a health authority withholding a treatment from a patient, the burden should be on the authority to explain why it has been withheld rather than on the individual to prove why it is needed. These ideas place the doctor–patient relationship at the centre of the debate.

Instead of choice, the service should be based around the involvement of the public in decision-making processes. The voice of users should be heard expressly throughout the service, saying what is wanted, rather than the mechanisms of choice determining what is needed.[18]

A council of experts

Doctors are growing increasingly restive, as we have seen. But, interestingly, the Royal College of Physicians produced a paper effectively advocating the utilitarian cause, suggesting priorities must be set at a national level and advocating a national council for health care priorities, which should monitor how health care priorities are set, allow open discussion, taking into account cost implications, setting parameters for health authorities to operate within, and incorporating the best evidence-based practice. Such a system could work from the bottom up – with doctors putting forward their experience of how treatments best worked, and allowing them to become more directly involved in the priority-setting process.[19]

A clear division of powers

Another way forward has been suggested by New and Le Grand. The individual's need for health services is unpredictable. There is the problem of information imbalance, with which we are familiar. In addition, health is of fundamental importance to other parts of life.[20]

But there has been extreme difficulty encountered by other systems in drawing up lists. And attempts to ration could undermine the security, solidarity and serenity that have been such important products of the system, and which have done so much to underpin its popularity.

Nonetheless, there is a need to be more rational about rationing. Even a list of those services that satisfy the three criteria above would still probably be too long and rationing would still be needed. This would have to be carried out by clinicians making decisions on the basis of clinical need and cost effectiveness.

Of course, deciding which services fit these criteria will be subjective and will require extensive debate. This is why it is of central importance that well-tried methods for debating are incorporated within the body of the system.

Clinical discretion will remain – it is ingrained deeply within the culture of the system. Doctors are likely to continue rationing, as they have traditionally, on their perception of need. Thus monitoring and openness are crucial.

These different proposals all reflect different problems and prejudices. Professor Dworkin is American and his solution reflects this – increased privatization, as we have noted, would be extremely problematic elsewhere. The notion of a right to health care sounds good, but what would it mean? How would it be established, and in what body of law? How easy would it be to establish this without increasing the economic liability of the State well beyond its capacity to supply it?

Le Grand and New say their system is a mixture of principle and pragmatism. That, perhaps, is as much as can be expected within the current context of rationing. But change in the rest of the system can only create pressures for acting within a defined set of principles, as rationing becomes more and more obvious. There is a need at least to debate the methods by which rationing dilemmas can be tackled. The debate must be wide ranging and public, and it will, inevitably, touch on all elements of the health system.

Beyond rationing: rational priorities

The British system is seen both to have equitable and inequitable tendencies. On the one hand, because it is funded through taxes it tends to redistribute resources from the rich to the poor. On the other it can be seen to be inequitable in the distribution of health care. Poor people are still found to be iller than rich people and the amount of extra spending they receive is not proportional to how ill they are.[21]

These are long-term issues, and they have posed problems for health secretaries for decades. In 1976 an attempt was made to adjust resource allocation in line with the populations of regions according to their age and sex. Since then, the resource allocation working party (RAWP) formula has worked to ensure more equitable allocation of resources. There have been criticisms of the RAWP approach – that it concentrated only on inputs to the health service and not on outputs, its crude use of mortality rates, its neglect of social deprivation indicators and its insensitivity to variations beneath the regional level. The RAWP formula has been replaced by a new formula. There have, however, been serious concerns voiced that this has increased the inequities in the system: the top ten gainers of this change are all south-eastern health authorities, the losers are mainly in northern industrial areas – a pattern, as one commentator has pointed out, tied in closely with the previous electoral strategy.[22]

There are also social inequalities built into the system as analysis of rates of heart disease and stroke have shown – professionals tend to suffer less than others, and much less than unskilled workers.[23]

According to a classic study by Julian Tudor Hart, a GP working in Wales, those living in deprived areas are less likely to have access to and to use health services than those in affluent areas. This he calls the 'inverse care law', and although the study is more than 25 years old, it is still widely respected.[24]

The problem was not a high priority in the previous Government's policy, despite the publication in 1996 of a report under the Health of the Nation initiative acknowledging the problems. The report states 'Studies in the UK have reported increasing socio-economic differentials in mortality, acknowledging the access to and use of health services ... along with environmental differences were among the causes of variation.' It pointed to ways the Department of Health and the NHS should work towards shifting the differences, with purchasers incorporating strategies for reducing inequalities by ensuring there is access to services for everyone.[23]

The document reviews much of the evidence for inequalities in health on geographical and social bases. It also makes clear that both the Department of Health and the NHS have local roles to play. The NHS has the tasks of identifying health variations at local level, setting targets for 'improving the health experience of particular groups or areas', providing effective access to health care services, involving a wide range of bodies in strategic alliances to improve health, allocating resources, initiating public health programmes aimed at individuals or groups, and acting as a responsible employer. GPs are required to have a plan for identifying and tackling interventions in co-ordination with other health bodies. GPs and trusts should also make sure there is equitable access to services in their areas.

The document displays many of the blame-dispersal techniques we noted in the Government's attitude to rationing. It is easy to see here the potential for acceptance by the Department and the Government of credit for the attack on inequity in the NHS, while making sure that the NHS itself can be blamed for any actual inequities that take place. The power to do this in the latter case is implicit in the second specific recommendation from the Department of Health. The strategy states: 'We recommend specifically that health authorities and GP purchasers should have a plan for identifying and tackling variations, and for evaluating interventions.'

The document represented the first direct look at inequalities in health produced by Government since the Black Report. It came as part of the Health of the Nation strategy in which 27 targets were chosen to encourage health promotion – including cutting coronary heart disease, cancers, dealing with mental illness, AIDS and keeping down the number of accidents.

On the face of it the impact of the Health of the Nation has been dramatic; targets have been met. Like the Patient's Charter, however, there is doubt about the targets themselves and the impact of other forces. The late incorporation of the inequalities in health document into the strategy shows that it missed a key – perhaps the key – point about health promotion in the NHS, namely, that if resources are going to be spent on public health, they should look to remedy inequalities, not increase them. It is the same logic as rationing and should set the framework within which decisions are taken. Perhaps the belated admission of inequality is the first condition for a more rational discussion about rationing itself.

References

1 Klein R (1993) Dimensions of rationing: who should do what? *BMJ*. **307**: 309–11.
2 Powell JE (1975) *Medicine and Politics*. (2nd ed.) Pitman Medical, London.
3 Mullen P (1995) *Is Healthcare Rationing Really Necessary?* Health Services Management Centre, Birmingham.
4 Hunter D (1993) *Rationing Dilemmas in Healthcare*. NAHAT, Birmingham.
5 Interview with Consultant Surgeon, London, September 1996.
6 Interview with Sir Duncan Nichol, October 1996.
7 Harrison S and Hunter D (1994) *Rationing Health Care*. Institute for Public Policy Research, London.
8 Redmayne S (1996) *Small Steps, Big Goals: purchasing policies in the NHS*. NAHAT, Birmingham; Klein R, Redmayne S and Day P (1993) *Sharing Out Resources: purchasing and priority setting in the NHS*. NAHAT, Birmingham.
9 For discussions of these processes see New B and Le Grand J (1996) *Rationing in the NHS: principles and pragmatism*. King's Fund, London; Klein R, Day P and Redmayne S (1996) *Managing Scarcity, Priority Setting and Rationing in the National Health Service*. Open University, Buckingham.
10 Bowling A (1996) Healthcare rationing: the public's debate. *BMJ*. **307**: 670–3.
11 Interview with Sir Michael Peckham, July 1996.
12 Mooney G and Olsen JA (1991) QALYs, where next?, in A Mcintyre (ed.) *Providing Healthcare: the economics of alternative systems*. OUP, Oxford.
13 Honigsbaum F, Calltorp J, Holmström S et al. (1995) *Priority Setting Processes for Healthcare*. Radcliffe Medical Press, Oxford; Honigsbaum F, Holmström S and Calltorp J (1997) *Making Choices for Healthcare*. Radcliffe Medical Press, Oxford.
14 There is a vast amount of press material covering the Child B case, see for example Toynbee P (1996) Jaymee and final choices: the story behind the story. *Independent*. May 23; Leader (1996) When rights collide: Jaymee's to fight, the NHS's to resist. *Guardian*. 23 May. See also Klein R, Redmayne S and Day P (1996) *Op Cit*.
15 Interviews with managers of Somerset Health Authority, Greater Glasgow Health Board and Bromley Health, 1996.
16 *A service with ambitions: the record of the NHS*, speech by Stephen Dorrell at a NAHAT symposium, 14 November 1996.
17 Smith R (1996) Being creative about rationing. *BMJ*. **312**: 391–2.
18 Lenaghan J (1996) *Rationing and Rights in Healthcare*. Institute for Public Policy Research, London; IPPR (1995) *Hard Choices in Healthcare: patients' rights and public priorities in the UK and Europe*. Institute for Public Policy Research, London.
19 Royal College of Physicians of London (1995) *Setting Priorities in the NHS: a framework for decision making*. RCP, London.
20 New B and Le Grand J (1996) *Op Cit*.
21 Wagstaff A, van Doorslaer E and Paci P (1989) Equity in the finance and delivery of health care: some tentative cross-country comparisons. *Oxford Review of Health Policy*. **5**(1): 89–112.

22 *Table manners at the healthcare feast: the case for spending less and getting more from the NHS*, speech by Alan Maynard at London School of Economics, 26 October 1995.

23 DoH (1996) *Health of the nation: Variations in health – what can the Department of Health and the National Health Service Do?* HMSO, London.

24 Tudor Hart J (1971) The inverse care law. *Lancet.* i: 405–12.

10 Conclusion: who cares?

We are dazzled by the present. The battles that run through the health system and which make the headlines every day – between consultants and hospital executives, between purchasers and providers, the admonition of politicians from Westminster and the cacophony of local MPs faced by threatened hospitals – block out the future. Living today, surviving until tomorrow is what matters. Next week, next year, is a different problem.

The British health debate is long on prognoses of doom, far shorter on visions for the future. The problems appear depressingly cyclical: the crisis facing the NHS last winter was one that has faced it since before the reforms. The problems of 1998 seem alarmingly familiar to those of 1988. Behind the headlines the pressures of demography, technology and consumer expectation point only one way – to high medical inflation and to demand that will outstrip supply. The system has coped in the past and may well cope in the future, but there is no room for complacency. Indeed, if the past ten years have illustrated anything, it is that the failure to take hard choices postpones, but does not ease, high pressure issues. It may be that the broadly nationalized system will be intact in 50 years' time, but it would be a brave man who bet on it retaining the basic features to which it has clung sentimentally for its first 50.

Where we have come from

The NHS was founded on a consensus that placed an autonomous medical profession at the centre, buttressed by clinical freedom, operating within a budgetary framework set out by central Government, itself interpreting the parameters of public opinion. Other agents – hospital and health authority administrators – held supporting roles.

The consensus was all embracing. Complex ethical decisions were made consensually. Broad economic decisions on priority setting were the preserve of Government and health authority. Deciding who shall live and who shall die, or at least who shall wait, was in the hands of the doctor. Doctors were prepared to take on the role as rationers of public health care in return for the deal struck at the outset of the service. It seemed a natural role for them to play – interpreting demand in terms of medical need. In the days of consensus it did not seem necessary, or indeed wise, to point out that the same personnel did not have to make decisions to treat on the same criteria in the private sector. There they were merely responding to paid-up demand, without the need to decide whether it was worthy of public finance.

Thus, traditionally, decision making has been obscured in the various groups within the health system. There may have been fundamental questions asked about whether or not the system was affordable – questions such as those raised by the Guillebaud Commission in the 1950s. There may have been developments that seemed to call into question the very principles of the service – such as the introduction of prescription charges, and charges for eye tests. But the context of these developments was still one of consensus, of the need to find ways to preserve the system.

Conservative reform from 1979 posed new questions. First, it asked 'Do we want a National Health Service?' 'Ought we to have one?' These questions never escaped the tightly controlled NHS review of 1987 within which, it was clear, some argued that the NHS should be gradually privatized. But politics dictated the answers to the two questions – 'yes' and 'yes'. Fundamental issues about the funding of the system – 'Should we spend more?' 'Should we spend less?' 'What financial mechanisms should be in place?' – were swept away with these answers. As a consequence efforts turned to living within the nationalized settlement and the broad financial landscape that had existed since 1948, squeezing more efficiency out of an inefficient system. This supply-side view accepted that the difficult choices – bringing doctors to heel for their spending decisions, rationing, making hospitals more efficient – would be perpetuated but, in theory at least, instead of allowing them to exist consensually, they would be taken ever more openly and accountably. The engine for this change was to be the market.

The logic flowing from reform also brought about a new need for openness, knowledge and information. The consensus was unquestioning. With Griffiths, reform opened a Pandora's box simply by asking who was in charge. The significance of this question, and of the nerve Griffiths and Thatcher had in asking it, would in theory see the compromise of consensus tumble like dominoes in the face of a tide of information and measurement. From this simple beginning would flow accountability, management, patient empowerment, and efficiency – without sacrificing equity. But the theories of reform could make little headway against the medical consensus. There may be a new structure to the system, but the goals of reform are still far away. There is information but it is often the wrong sort. The acceptance of the hybrid 'contestability' indicates that interest groups have been too powerful for the logic of management and market to overcome entirely, despite changing the way in which different elements of the system operated, and related to, one another.

Where to now?

If the NHS is to be here in 50 years' time, a new start is needed. The blueprint of reform had little respect for consensus and squeezed out the voice of public users and professionals in managing the system, preferring 'choice' to 'voice'. Ironically, as we have seen, this is one fundamental reason why it has failed to achieve what it set out to do.

The problems addressed in this book – medical unaccountability, ineffi-cient resource allocation, inequity, lack of clarity on financing, the need for rational hospital reconfiguration, for rational practice and a rational profession, and for rational and fair rationing – are scarcely more advanced than they were in 1983 or even 1987. There is a new structure that can theoretically engineer change, but there has been little political, and even less medical, will to see it happen.

A new, inclusive idiom is needed with which the structure can be used to bring about change. There is a need for far greater debate on the issues of health and the prevailing listlessness is reinforced by the lack of a national conversation. What narrow channels for debate there were have dried up in the centralization of the system that we noted in Chapters 4 and 5. What exists now is a monologue that has undermined the ability of the British people to examine their system and be a part of it. If discus-sion about the service continues to be muted can we expect people to be interested? There are some hard choices to be made, but unless they are made quickly the NHS will die a slow death as its credibility as a national system is undermined. Taken together, what is proposed here may seem radical, even extreme, but it is less extreme than the alternative – allowing the NHS to rot away, leaving our children with nothing.

Pressing questions

What future for the market?

The failure of the market was a wasted opportunity. As was argued in Chapter 3, the metaphor was misconceived, exposing the Government to accusations that it was setting the system up for privatization. What is proposed by the Government now maintains the strengths of the market system – the analytical framework of the purchaser/provider split – while tinkering with the problems under the guise of abolition. In the long term this will not do. It may be the case that an overly competitive market is inappropriate for the health system, particularly in the public sector. However the move towards five-year contracting periods is emphasizing the wrong solution to the right problem. Contracting lies at the root of market failure, both undermining effective analysis through the purchaser/provider split and ruling out effective competition. It will remain so unless contracts with meaningful information about what is being paid for and provided by the taxpayer come about, and that means ending the dominance of block contracting. Information, not the timescale, is the key to efficiency.

This has serious implications for much of what follows. Accountability can only be ensured through information. The growing desire of the public – and for their proxies, the purchasers and GP fundholders – to see clearly what it is spending its money on – the argument for hypothecating taxation – requires not only macroeconomic signals but hard microeconomic information to which those signals relate; otherwise they are meaningless. A rational rationing system can never come about unless it is clear what commissioners or purchasers intend to spend their money on. Hospitals cannot be reconfigured unless what they do and how much it costs is known. Doctors' performance cannot be measured without anything to measure. In the absence of information that means something, how can anyone expect the health system to change for the better?[1]

Doctors and patients

The most fundamental problem is the relationship between doctor and patient. It is here where the culture against information is born. Traditionally, doctors act as agents for patients because of the catastrophic effects of illness and because of the problems of information imbalance. What, in short, is the use of information – on clinical conditions, on treatments, on cost effectiveness – if patients and the public cannot relate it to anything they understand? From this starting point a whole culture of immeasurability is built.

This mindset must change. The balance of knowledge must be shifted towards the patient in future. It is a complex proposition because in many cases patients may not seek greater knowledge or wish for increased responsibility. They may wish for solace in the consulting-room chair. In addition, despite the visions of John Spiers and Adam Darkins, the information imbalance is unlikely to be overturned completely, and may be shifted in different degrees for different people and different conditions.[2]

Nevertheless, one forward-thinking doctor believes that the medical model of health is under threat as society becomes less certain of what doctors can actually deliver. The combination of conditions like AIDS and TB which has rocked confidence, along with the rise of alternative therapies, is changing the way patients think about medicine. As Harrison writes:

> Even though, or perhaps because, these therapies are not sufficiently scientifically proven, their popularity appears to be on the increase. They offer something new, and potentially liberating, with different sets of rules operating between therapist and client, when compared with more traditional doctor–patient dynamics.[3]

Instead of a relationship of dominance, there could be greater partnership between doctors and patients in future. The unbalanced relationship has undermined attempts to create an accountable system because there is little understanding between the people who use the system, and those who provide it, about what is being done. If the possibility of understanding was accepted, the whole status of information would be changed. Patients could expect more information on their condition and to be able to enter meaningful discussions with doctors. But fundamental change must happen outside the doctor's surgery and the public must ask what it expects of doctors. It cannot, on the one hand, have gatekeepers and guardians of their tax liability for the NHS in times of health and on the other have a Hippocratic, individually-focused medic attending to every need in times of sickness. The confidentially-based, individually-focused doctor may have been incorporated within the post-war system but, as we have seen, economic fortune has waned, medical costs have soared and we just can't afford what once we could.

It is here where the nature of the problem appears overwhelming. How can we reconcile the irreconcilable – the duty to the individual and the duty to the community? These are ethical positions that can only exist in conflict – hence the extent of conflict within the system.

The doctor's responsibility to his patient and to society needs to be set in a new framework. Since the necessity for doing this is underpinned by the stewardship of public funds, the public ought to have a say in redrawing the position. Members of the public need to be asked what they expect of the doctor both in their capacity as patients and as citizens.

One concept that has been used throughout the history of the service is the charter. In the 1960s Kenneth Robinson's GPs Charter illustrated the medical dominance in the system. In the 1990s, it was the turn of the patient to have a charter. The new Government proposes a charter itself which could have dramatic effect if it is permitted a radical agenda. The new charter should seek to establish the relationship between the doctor and patient at an individual level, and between medicine and society on a wider scale. A good starting point would be the scrapping of the Hippocratic oath, which buttresses the refusal of doctors to acknowledge their socio-economic role as of any importance alongside their medical one with centuries of mystique and tradition. Such a charter should be placed within a context of, and run parallel to, a national debate on other crucial issues such as what the health service should be for, how services should be rationed, what hospitals should do, how people should be treated. It should also underpin a new accountability, forged on partnership. The method of the charter, delivered through every door in the country, was used in 1991. The letter box, e-mail address and website could and should be used to invigorate debate.

Accountability

We have discussed at length the ways in which the individual is perceived in relation to the health system. We have seen that making the responsibilities of patients clear as well as their rights, is crucial to the understanding of how the health system can flourish in future.

Giving the consumer choice, making the service more responsive, breaking the power of producer interests have all been a part of the philosophy of reform. They have been limited by the lack of choice within the market – choice of GP, of health authority, of hospitals and doctors – and limited by the structure of the market and the lack of contestability in some areas. They have also been limited by the power of the medical profession to resist change and by the fact that the patient cannot consume in the health marketplace as he does in Sainsbury's.

Although information can be used to help patients and the public in their role as citizens, the distortions caused by imposing a commercial model on a public service like the NHS has meant the public has been frozen out of the dialogue. Where interest groups have fought to define their positions on the new battlefield of the health market, patients have been absent, unable to judge whether others are acting in their interests, or unable to make their own positions clear. Predicating a system on choice, when those who are supposed to do the choosing – or are having the choosing done for them – are in an extremely vulnerable position may be wrong headed. Vulnerability may undermine the ability to make rational choices. This is particularly the case when the vulnerable can only express preferences on which a choice is made by the doctor.

Nevertheless, the reconceptualization of the old system as a market has gone some way to achieving what it set out to do – it has begun to let us see how to contain the costs of that system. In the purchaser/provider split it has created a much more powerful framework on which the dynamics, relationships and costs of the system can be analysed. It has tried to make the system more pluralistic in a commercial sense, by making a contestable marketplace of buyers and sellers across the public and private sectors. As we have noted, it has fallen short. But can it be taken further?

The answer, surely, is yes. It lies in more sensitive information – as suggested above. But it also depends on allowing the concepts of participation – of 'voice' in Hirschman's formulation – to be married with those of 'exit'. We noted earlier in the chapter how one great tension in the new system was the need for openness and the blocking of channels of expression and accountability at local level. The market system permitted one form of pluralism – choice which did not function as planned – but has quashed another – debate.[4] This has happened against a background of devolving decision making into local contexts while accountability is exercised only from the centre. This is too weak.

As Anna Coote makes clear, the public 'is deeply interested in health and illness', but 'the actual connection between the public and policy making on health is negligible'. Coote points out that there is a lack of accountability in the system – both in the ability of local people to hold the bodies taking decisions that directly effect them to account, and in the information that is given out by those bodies to account for their decisions. Decision making has been devolved down the pyramid of the system, to the grass roots in the case of the GP fundholder, while accountability has been concentrated at the pinnacle – with the Government and the Secretary of State.[5]

The reform process has stifled debate. We have seen how health authorities, trusts, CHC and GP fundholders are unaccountable to the public and how CHCs have no rights of representation on the boards of health bodies and operate with tiny budgets. None of these models tends towards the involvement of the public in deciding how health services should be provided and what resources should be put into them.

The limitations of the public in the consumer model could be made good by incorporating them into the decision-making one. There are two ways of doing this. We have noted the lack of accountability of health bodies and the need to open them up to scrutiny and Government initiatives here are positive. Mechanisms for bringing local representation on to the boards of health authorities should be re-examined. One possibility is to reintroduce the local authority members. Another could be to boost CHCs and their funding, and bring CHC members on to health authorities. A third, more radical, option could be to turn health purchasing over to local authorities – as may happen in post-devolution Scotland – which would combine the legitimacy of election to health authorities with the integration of health into other areas of public policy. All of these options should be considered and piloted.

There are, however, concerns about representation and legitimacy. One is that the public is too lethargic to care. This is where focus groups can play a significant part. We have already examined how a citizens' jury in Walsall debated the options for palliative care and was able to engage in complicated and sophisticated arguments.[6] Focus groups should continue to be used as and when they are considered necessary, but it is worth noting that the motivation for calling on a jury – and paying over the money to have one set up – is to add legitimacy to decision making, a legitimacy that is lacking in the current system. As Michael Evans made clear in the previous chapter, the citizens' jury not only enhanced accountability – it was also able, to his surprise, to enhance the quality of its decision making.

These principles justify a wider use of such mechanisms. The citizens' jury could be broadened to add powerful local opinion at a given time in the contracting cycle, and incorporated into purchasing plans. It may have a larger membership, take in other agencies and take longer to examine the issues thrown up by a purchasing plan, but it would call doctors and managers as witnesses and have a formalized relationship with health authorities or commissioning groups, which would have to incorporate its recommendations into its purchasing plans or explain why they had not been incorporated. As we have seen, these decisions could be set within the context of a national body, such as the one suggested by the Royal College of Physicians.[7]

One other key concern about opening up the accountability of the system is the cost. Citizens' juries and focus groups are expensive. A budget should be made available to health authorities for consultation, and the mechanisms for consultation should not exceed this.

These processes of drawing a greater spectrum of opinion into the decision making of the system will make explicit not only what is going to be delivered by the NHS, but what the public expects it to deliver. Debates would be conducted within a context of the greater understanding of the tradeoffs between the individual and the social. The two elements would be perceived as opposing parts of a whole – similar to the mechanisms of choice and voice that would operate together, the one constraining the other.

For a system of accountability to work the doctors themselves have to be open to greater accountability. A starting point would be to ensure the planned structures of accountability are made effective. This means closer scrutiny of contracting among GP fundholders and commissioning groups as well as health authorities to ensure they are being implemented properly and achieving value for money. Commissioners must consult the public and make clear what their purchasing strategies are.

Within hospitals those tools of management that have been put in place – like job plans – must be made effective. This does not mean managers crash in heavy handedly to impose unwanted regimes on defensive doctors. As one pilot in Oxford has shown, working patterns can be made more efficient and open just as well by doctors as by managers. The ideal must be to bring management and clinical staff together, as Jenny Simpson of BAMM argues.[8] Changes in outdated contract, pay and time allocation are best managed together but there has to be acceptance that change is needed.

It is clear that the audit measures that have been introduced since the 1990 reforms have gone some way, but by no means far enough, in bringing accountability to bear. Information should be part of a strengthening of the relationship between managers and doctors. We have seen how doctors' contracts give them the freedom to decide at what level they wish to pitch the guarantee of security within the NHS. They can choose to have all their income guaranteed by the State, or a part of it, calculating how much they will be able to earn in the private sector and matching this to what they require from the NHS. It is desirable to have a private sector within the system – although operating within a clearer set of guidelines than at present – and the contract system fits well within that broader aim. However, the tools for ensuring contracts are followed are weak. We have seen how job plans have been implemented patchily, and the work plans of junior doctors even more so. There is still a great deal of autonomy in the way doctors work. This may be the preferred option of management – regarding it no more important to keep traditionally autonomous doctors happy than to spell out the exact limitations of that autonomy.

A change in culture is needed. Management can only be effective if the tools at its disposal are widely accepted. It is true that management cannot work in the health service as it does in industry – doctors will always need some freedom to make clinical decisions. But the parameters of those decisions must be made clear to managers, just as the basis for the relationship between doctor, patient and society is made clear through a new charter. If the doctors of the future are going to fit into an accountable framework, measures like job plans have to gain acceptance.

This should not shackle doctors into rigid, monotonous, initiativeless working patterns. Doctors must maintain input into their working condi-

tions and the parameters of what they do. The breaking down of professional barriers could and ought to have a lot to do with introducing a
challenging and dynamic working environment for doctors, but it must,
as we noted in Chapter 8, be overseen properly. This is where a co-operative and respectful relationship between management and clinical staff
must be established.

Professional practice, effectiveness and quality

Information on doctors' performance is thin. This is an extremely sensitive
area, but it is one that has to be tackled if the system is to make sense.
Some form of accountability over the actions of doctors is needed,
although there are limitations in both practical and ideal senses.

The protestations of Dr Macara make it clear how much resistance and
fear there is by doctors to having information about individual outcomes
being made available. The ability of Dr Harry Burns in Glasgow to get
doctors to accept compromise protocols was down to him making clear to
what use he would put such information.[9] However, the reluctance of
doctors to have their performance accounted for is based on a conception
of the use the information would be put to. The feeling is that it would be
used as a stick to beat doctors, but, as Dr Burns makes clear, the more
information there is the more opportunity there is for coming to agreements on how to improve performance.

The opposition to allowing more information to become available is
clothing secrecy in the spurious legitimacy of confidentiality. We have
seen how increased information is the key to sustaining support for the
present system; indeed it may be the only way of justifying it. This is
crucial for doctors. One of the key factors of the breakdown in the old
order of health care is an erosion of the respect for the medical profession.
The public are now more questioning than ever about the abilities of
doctors and their right to be unaccountable. Coupled with the wider need
for greater information, resistance by doctors to greater scrutiny can only
create greater pressure.

Dr Macara has made it clear that the doctors' support for the limited
auditing procedures that have been accepted so far has been as much out
of the self-interest of a traditional interest group as through anything else,
but still he and the profession hold out against outcomes information.
Despite the fact that this reluctance to allow outcomes appears like a
rearguard action, the importance of context in the provision of information is fundamental. While it seems unreasonable of Macara to suggest
that the complexity of figures on medical performance would make them

incomprehensible to the layman, it is also unreasonable to expect the medical profession immediately to accept the publication of outcomes figures in the pages of the daily newspapers. Some compromise must be reached.

The information ought to be available in a system that has been predicated on the patient. The rhetoric of rights has been used in the Patient's Charter. Surely, if the health service is to operate over the next 50 years, we cannot believe that patients are passively going to continue to accept that they should be prevented from knowing whether the person cutting them up or prescribing a course of treatment for them has a good track record? If the health system is to be re-established for the new millennium, surely this kind of information is crucial to its credibility?

One suggestion has been to boost the power of the Confidential Enquiry into Peri-operative Deaths. Brendan Devlin, as we have seen, argues that the confidential part should be dropped. Others have suggested that the enquiry should be put under the direction of the Audit Commission, which would continue it as an ongoing audit of the standards of the medical profession. The enquiry would then pass from the status of a self-regulating mechanism into a statutory one. There seems logic to this, since the doctors are technically employed by the State. But again, there would have to be safeguards against the misuse of the information.[10]

If the information, with context and casemix etc. was made available to health authorities it could then be used by managers to measure performance and to influence purchasing decisions. The same information could be made available to GP fundholders, and commissioning groups to make the same decisions. This would provide information that is currently lacking in the operation of the market. Alongside types of contract that contain better information – more cost and volume instead of block – the relationships between purchasers and providers, which are here to stay, as we have seen, could be made much more realistic and operate on a sounder footing.

Alongside changes in working conditions must come changes in clinical practice. The arguments for evidence-based medicine have been rehearsed in previous chapters. Here it suffices to say that EBM fits exactly within the spirit of a new, information-driven system. People have as much right to know that the treatment being carried out on them is as effective as the doctor performing it. The new National Institute for Clinical Excellence could be a powerful tool in this. However, EBM should not be oversold. It is no panacea – as some of the enthusiastic publications of political parties suggest. There will continue to be rationing while ineffective treatments are being weeded out of the system and while waste is being dispatched along with them. It may be that rationing will continue after this – indeed it is difficult to conceive of a system without rationing. The Government's moves towards quality indicators are a step in the right direction. They must defend them.

Financing

The funding question has been dodged in favour of supply-side reform, but as in other areas of the system, openness can be the only way forward. We saw in Chapter 6 how increasingly discerning consumers were less willing to see their money wasted in inefficient public services, and were therefore ever more vigilant over tax levels. On the other hand we saw how it was unwilling to see services, particularly high profile ones like the NHS, in decline. The logical implication of these factors is to give people more information about what their money is going on. Short of a full pricing system, that information is always going to be approximate.

However, there are two ways in which this information could and should be integrated into NHS care. First, health expenditure should be hypothecated for the reasons set out above. Second, there should be charges for elements of the system – 'hotel' and non-clinical services for example. The level of charges and the question of means testing and grading them to ensure they are not regressive should be matters of public debate. The charges should be made only for secondary care – primary care should remain free at the point of use in order not to discourage preventative health care. Third, and alongside these developments, debate on the level of health spending should be encouraged. Do we want to increase our spending up to European levels? What would we want extra money spent on – reducing waiting, lists, bricks and mortar, universalization of gene therapy?

These questions are of major importance and until they are answered no clear view on the future of the system can be taken, and no long-term strategy setting out which part of it is set out to do what can be formulated. There are implications in this for the private sector, which are considered below. Without tackling the mechanisms of financing it is impossible to resolve the dilemma that in a system without prices there is little hope of controlling demand. A more transparent system could create a much more viable horizon of responsibility.

It is a truism to say that demand will always outstrip supply as long as there are no prices to control it, but beyond this it is possible to qualify and analyse to a greater extent one the parameters of the system are more widely understood. Making the supply side of the system better and more efficient without questioning the financing will only encourage demand,

and we fall into the vicious circle outlined by Professor Nick Bosanquet. The NHS becomes a victim of its own success. As it concentrates ever more on becoming efficient it becomes less equitable, less fair. As it becomes less fair it loses support for the methods of allocating resources that must accompany such a public system – priority setting and rationing. Once it begins to lose support for what was seen to be the very reason for it being set up, its days are numbered. Its success has destroyed it.

For Bosanquet the answer is a partnership scheme which, he argues, introduces the disciplines of a pricing mechanism without destroying the public service ethos. Faced with the modern needs of disease management and chronic illness, partnership schemes may offer a practical method of dealing with the costs of the future. If such a scheme is piloted in long-term care it will be worth following its progress carefully.[11]

Hospital reconfiguration

Similar techniques could be used to deal with reconfiguration of services. The current framework within which these critical decisions are taken is *ad hoc* and easily manipulated, as the experience of Jill Turner shows.[12] Again, the quality of debate could be strengthened by the more fundamental discussions that would take place in redefining the doctor's role in the system.

Reconfiguration issues have fundamental implications for health spending. The flow of money through the system, decisions on where we should be treated, by whom, when and for how long, all have considerable impacts on resources. The old answers – in hospital, by a consultant, as soon as possible and for ages – may no longer be affordable. Again, the debate on the place of the individual in the context of society will be better understood by patients who have been invited to think and discuss the issues with doctors.

The Government has made it clear that it is to look again at hospital reconfiguration within London. Its appointment of a physician to head the new enquiry – 'Tomlinson II' – may or may not be an indication of the kinds of answers it expects on the closure of Barts and so on. It is clear that a similar exercise is needed around the country as the DGHs of the 1962 hospital plan look ever more like white elephants. More work is needed on the requirements for local hospitals throughout the country and some of this may be done within the announced health action zones. To maintain a semblance of equity, however, these initiatives need to be rolled out more fully. It is important that communities are involved in the decision making and integrated with management of the new institutions which emerge.

More work also needs to be done on the internal dynamics of hospitals, cost effectiveness, economies of scale, equality of access, the scope and range of services on offer, and the safety, economy and acceptability of community-based alternatives to hospital care. It is clear that reconfiguration of hospital services has major implications for the financial status of the system. It is also clear that hospitals are a great deal easier to open than to close. A nationwide study and debate on the network could make it clearer to the public that the one must dictate a compromise over the other.

Rationing

Rationing of health care is the end result of scarcity, which itself will have been determined by the factors outlined above. One of the more ambitious expectations of the reforms was to make clear the rationing mechanisms that have accompanied British health care since it was nationalized. The purchaser/provider split would ensure that health authorities and fundholders made clear what they were going to buy and so reveal the pattern of rationing services that had always taken place behind closed doors.

As Klein has pointed out, this often amounted to little more than a 'dance of the veils', where greater openness is hinted at but not actually followed through. Authorities may claim to be brave in taking hard decisions, whereas in fact they are only stating that certain treatments are very low priority and handing over to doctors the hard decisions on who should have IVF treatment, or which over 65s should be deprived of haemodialysis and allowed to die. The situation has been compounded by the explicit statement of the Department of Health that no treatments should be ruled out entirely by any health authority. Thus Berkshire, which had dipped its toe into the icy rationing brook, withdrew it quickly before it was snapped off.[13]

If decisions are to be taken rationally, they must be taken consistently, within a legitimate and accountable framework. The basis for this lies in the redefinition of the doctor–patient relationship in a new charter and as this process revolves on asking the question 'what is a doctor?', the starting point for rationing issues is 'what is an illness?'. This is a question which lies at the basis of a society's attitude to its health system.

Defining what it considers to be an illness allows it to decide what to pay for and what to shift out of the public domain. As discussed in the last chapter, there are many questions that have to be encountered, but the debate will cause policymakers, the public, professionals and politicians to embrace the value-laden questions that should determine what a health system sets out to do.

There are, as we saw in Chapter 5, arguments for establishing patients' rights to health care. It is difficult to see what this could add to the present settlement – where the existence of the NHS suggests such a 'right', or at least the ability to access services, is already established – beyond creating more litigation by enshrining it in law. In addition, such a right would be demonstrably different in different parts of the country, and if it was used as a legal mechanism to correct inequities overnight it could compound the problem. Its meaning would also change over time, depending on what money was available.

Instead of a right, a less ambitious option of increased public involvement in the decision making of an imperfect system may move in the same direction. Within this new context, health authority and commissioning group purchasing plans can take on a new significance. Instead of being the dance of the veils characterized by Klein, they can begin to tackle the questions that purchasers seem keen to address. What is on the menu? Under what circumstances should treatments be withheld? What criteria are we to apply to the effectiveness of treatment? What circumstances can we envisage for allowing the rules to be bent in exceptional cases?

If the debate around a new health charter was serious, the starting point for discussion around these issues would not be so depressingly backward as it was in the case of Child B. Even within this new context, there needs to be more than a simple statement by health authorities of what their proposals are. Further methods of integrating opinion, legitimacy and accountability into the decision making could be envisaged. On the one hand the health authority itself could be opened up to the local population. On the other, the principles of focus groups during the discussion of citizens' juries could be applied.

Within this context the call by the Royal College of Physicians for a national council for priority setting makes sense. Here, broad ethical and economic considerations could be studied openly. There would clearly be theoretical and methodological difficulties – as similar experiments in Oregon, Holland and New Zealand have indicated – but instead of using these as an excuse for complacency, they should be used as starting points for an exploration of resource allocation challenges in the British context. All the factors listed throughout this book are currently bringing pressure to bear on rationing decisions. If they are resolved they may lessen the pressure on rationing, but they are unlikely ever to rid us of the need for it as demand is pushed ever higher. We need a clear debate and a solid framework if these decisions are to maintain legitimacy for themselves and underpin the system itself. 'Muddling through elegantly' means muddling through to oblivion as far as the NHS is concerned.

At a local level, the idea of the focus group incorporated into purchasing decisions will also inform rationing decisions. These must work with rejuvenated and accountable local agencies – health authorities, commissioning agencies, trusts and community health councils, primary care teams, patient groups and local democratic fora – starting with local authorities. These groups should be brought together specifically to discuss rationing at given times throughout the contracting cycle, constantly questioning and challenging the way resources are spent.

The question of equity would exist alongside the question of rationing. The existence of a national body would define the margins within which local decisions could be made. It would thus decide the extent of variation in treatment around the country – a variation that currently exists, as it has since 1948 – and make it explicit. Equity would be interpreted by each health authority in their decisions about how to relate themselves to criteria set out nationally, and therefore how they would relate to other areas. Of course, this would be acknowledging another taboo: that there *are* variations. But the suggestion that variations undermine the claims of the system to be national are overstated. A willingness to recast the national system around the variations that exist throughout the country would strengthen, not undermine, it.

Le Grand and New point to an explicit version of the system that currently exists – where the Government decides broad parameters and the doctors interpret them. By making it explicit, the system becomes legitimized by incorporating public values rather than operating behind closed doors, with every decision taken by doctor, politician or administrator. This is as good a starting point as any, but it could lead on to greater openness and clarity, as outlined above.[14]

Some practical indications of what is currently happening and where difficulties lie is given by Honigsbaum *et al.*, who point out that the only place where exclusion of treatment has been applied across the board is in Oregon – and that too has run into difficulties. In the UK rationing using guidelines has grown in use and this process could be encouraged, although it hands over power to doctors. It is possible, he says, to use guidelines within a framework of exclusions that feed in public opinion. This is another way of expressing Le Grand and New's division of powers, and it seems the most sensible way forward. Honigsbaum stresses, however, that this will be a slow and emergent process, and no big bang.[15]

Public and private sectors

Another unclear area that would be clarified by greater explicitness would be the relationship between the public and private sectors. We saw in previous chapters how the division between the two sectors is at best fluid, and at worst muddy. It makes it difficult both for private and public sectors to plan their services and be aware of whom they are aiming to take care of. The maintenance of the status quo acts as a disincentive for the private sector to look at regulating and improving its products. At the moment it acts in a space defined by the public perception of the NHS. Policy initiatives such as concentration on bringing down waiting lists would have major consequences for the private sector. The ability of trusts to compete with private sector providers by offering pay beds is also changing the relationship between the sectors.

These are not circumstances favourable to a rational system and they are not circumstances favourable to the private sector putting its house in order – as 1996's OFT report suggested it should.[16] The problems of small print, of policy exclusions, of not taking previous conditions, or moratorium underwriting would all clearly be unacceptable to organizations whose purpose was to provide a social service. There is a clear need to encourage the private sector to gear policies towards lifetime cover, rather than making them renewable annually, but the private sector can only be expected to change these practices to the extent to which it is accepted as a part of that social system. At the moment it is not. Greater precision about what the NHS is expected to do and what is beyond its remit would clarify the issue.

As we saw earlier, there are various options for defining the 'hinge' in the health system – the relationship between the public and private system. The current position is *ad hoc* but the logic in the British health system now points away from a consensus guaranteed by muddling through. Clarity is needed, and that points to the options suggested by Roderick Nye of the Social Market Foundation – a system used by some all of the time or all some of the time.[17]

Making those over a certain income opt out of the State system, receive a tax credit and buy their own insurance seems unfavourable because it divides society and it could lead to the undermining of support for the safety net system that would be left in place. Of course, the detail – at what level of income would an opt out be required – is important, but such a system would undermine a political objective – maintaining universal access for all – without necessarily solving the rationing problem: what should the NHS pay for? Making the NHS able to deal with demand by taking away a proportion of the users of the service seems an unsatisfactory and indirect way of dealing with the problem of deciding what is available through taxpayers' money. A clearer distinction could be made not by deciding who the NHS will treat, but what it will treat, attempting to maintain the system as inclusive of all people so that all people have an interest in seeing it work as best it can. It is here that we return to the redefinition of the health deal and of what the public can expect – to the fundamentals of the rationing dilemma outlined by New and Le Grand.[14]

Drawing lines is extremely difficult, but one way forward has been suggested by New and Le Grand:

> The boundary between what the NHS does and what other agencies do, or what individuals do for themselves is at present developing on *ad hoc* case law basis, and this cannot promote a sense of geographical equity, not a clear shared understanding of what the NHS should provide.

There is clearly a need to be more rational about rationing. We need to be clear about the kinds of services the NHS should provide. Of course, deciding what services fit these criteria will be subjective and will require extensive debate. Indeed, redefining the basis of the services provided by the NHS on any criteria will require debate. This is why it is of central importance that well-tried methods for debating are incorporated within the body of the system, why experimentation with focus groups, with conventions, with national priority setting bodies is needed.

With greater clarity arising from defining what services were available, decisions which could possibly be taken in future by local health conventions acting within the parameters set out by the national body on priority setting, there would be a clearer view of what services anyone could expect and what was to be paid for personally. A debate on tax relief on insurance premiums could then be conducted much more accurately. If reliefs were agreed, the level could be determined in relation to the extent of private, as opposed to state, coverage. These levels could fluctuate over time and would obviously not equate to 100% of premium prices – otherwise the redistribution in the tax system would be undermined along with its progressivity. However, such a system would allow the arguments over the equity or inequity inherent in the public/private mix to be followed with a great deal more clarity, where the debate now is too cumbersome.

Finally, let us return to the newborn daughter we left in Chapter 1. Looking ahead 50 years, that daughter was liberated by information. She was able to use the Internet to reach her own conclusions about the kinds of treatment she needed. She was able to exercise choice because she had knowledge. Her relationship with her doctor was one of much greater equality. The system she moved around was integrated – the term used by Dr Burns to describe the way a better functioning services should be designed – but she was the factor defining the integration.

Is this a viable future? People like John Spiers believe it is. They believe information technology can transform the power of patients to make choices for themselves, choices that will marginalize the arguments and frictions of the other interest groups in the service. They will be aligned around the need to serve the individual. Spiers believes the undercurrents of change are already with us, that information must sweep us into a future wholly different from the present:

> the most persuasive impact of new technologies is, of course, where it flows with those cultural shifts which already form a torrent. These are the torrents of greater international competition and transparency, and of greater self-reliance. Towards choice and liberty and away from dependence on professionals, away from myth, mystique and mystery.[18]

Spiers' conception of the use of technology fills one half of what the public can do for themselves in the world of health: choose. The other half is to shout. The notion of electronic democracy – virtual commissioning meetings – is as valid as that of technology bolstering information and freedom through choice. The two can work side-by-side, and there is no reason why your daughter should not have access to such a world.

Indeed, as information becomes available at lower levels, the possibilities of transparency become greater. The problems of excessive demand that dog the system could be placed within a context of greater understanding. It may be that showing people how much they pay into the system and how much they demand from it, may not be enough to slake demand for health care. The triumvirate of demand may continue to press upwards. However, it is possible that greater knowledge may at least enrich discussion about how much money is being spent on the system, and whether this is an appropriate level. Comparisons between private and public sectors – on a personal level as well as a national – would be easier to make. The notion of health care as a free good could be fundamentally questioned. The question 'Are you willing to pay more in tax for the health service?' would become a more meaningful one. Such transparency can only stimulate debate.

Hypothecation therefore could help break the problem of increased spending, merely revealing increased demand by linking in a sense of greater responsibility. This book has not set out to lay down definitive answers. It has argued instead that the most valuable goal we can set ourselves, perhaps the only one we can achieve, is to create the means to measure the system and to decide what we want from its various parts. The ethical decisions will change over time, and may vary with different emphases in different parts of the country. What we need to be clear about is how decisions are being taken and who is taking them. A sensible discussion can be had about the future demands to be placed on the system and how to meet them. At present, there is so little debate that despite recent white papers, the system seems to be wandering listlessly towards the new millennium without a clear course and without a clear mandate from the public. There is a need for clarity of purpose and direction. The time for a fundamental debate on its future has come. It is a debate of great importance and one we must face now, before it is too late.

References

1 See Spiers J (1995) *The Invisible Hospital and the Secret Garden: an insider's commentary on the NHS reforms.* Radcliffe Medical Press, Oxford, pp. 120–30.
2 Spiers J (1997) *Who Owns Our Bodies? making moral choices in health care.* Radcliffe Medical Press, Oxford; Darkins A (1996) *Shared Decision Making in Health Care Systems: working paper.* Unpublished.
3 Harrison J (1998) *The GP Tomorrow: living with uncertainty.* Radcliffe Medical Press, Oxford.
4 Hirschman A (1970) *Exit, Voice and Loyalty: responses to decline in firms, organizations and states.* Harvard University Press, Cambridge, MA.
5 Coote A (1997) The democratic deficit, in M Marinker (ed.) *Sense and Sensibility in Health Care.* BMJ Publishing Group, London.
6 Interview with Walsall Citizens' Jury, August 1996.
7 Royal College of Physicians of London (1995) *Setting Priorities in the NHS: a framework for decision making.* RCP, London.
8 Simpson J (1995) Managing the relationship between doctors and managers, in K Holdaway (ed.) *The Healthcare Management Handbook.* Kogan Page, London; Simpson J (1994) Doctors in management: dream or nightmare. *Proceedings of the Royal College of Physicians of Edinburgh.* 24: 197–202.
9 Interviews with Dr Sandy Macara, July 1996; Dr Harry Burns, August 1996.
10 Maynard A (1996) Health: a matter of facts. *Health Service Journal.*
11 Bosanquet N (1995) *Public Spending into the Millennium.* Social Market Foundation, London.
12 Turner J (1994) *Current Issues in Acute Care I: reconfiguring acute services.* Institute of Health Services Management, London; Turner J (1995) *Current Issues in Acute Care: reconfiguring acute services II.* Institute of Health Services Management, London; Turner J (1996) *Current Issues in Acute Care: reconfiguring acute services III.* Institute of Health Services Management, London.
13 Klein R, Day P and Redmayne S (1996) *Managing Scarcity, Priority Setting and*

Rationing in the National Health Service. Open University Press, Buckingham; Berkshire Health Commission (1996) *Purchasing Plan 1996/97.*

14 New B and Le Grand J (1996) *Rationing in the NHS: principles and pragmatism.* King's Fund, London.

15 Honigsbaum F, Holmström S and Calltorp J (1997) *Making Choices for Healthcare.* Radcliffe Medical Press, Oxford.

16 Office of Fair Trading (1996) *Health Insurance.* OFT, London.

17 Interview with Roderick Nye, November 1995.

18 Spiers J (1997) *Op Cit.*

Index